EVERYTHING YOU NEED TO KNOW

A Patient's Guide to Knee and Hip Replacement

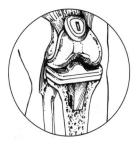

IRWIN SILBER

FOREWORD BY
EUGENE M. WOLF, M.D.

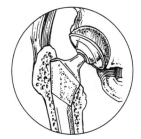

A FIRESIDE BOOK
Published by Simon & Schuster

This book is intended to provide helpful information about joint-replacement surgery. It is sold with the understanding that the author and the publisher are not engaged in rendering medical services in the book. Joint-replacement surgery, like all major surgery, requires careful consultation with competent medical professionals.

The author and the publisher specifically disclaim all responsibility for any liability, loss, or risk, personal or otherwise, incurred as a consequence, directly or indirectly, of the use and application of any of the contents of this book.

Questions or comments to the author or Dr. Wolf can be addressed to Dr. Wolf's web site: www.eugene-wolf-md.com.

F

FIRESIDE
Rockefeller Center
1230 Avenue of the Americas
New York, NY 10020

Illustration credits appear on page 241.

FIRESIDE and colophon are registered trademarks of Simon & Schuster Inc.

Designed by Jenny Dossin
Manufactured in the United States of America
10 9 8 7 6 5 4 3 2 1

Library of Congress Cataloging-in-Publication Data
Silber, Irwin, date.
    A patient's guide to knee and hip replacement : everything you need to know / Irwin Silber ; foreword by Eugene M. Wolf.
        p.   cm.
"A Fireside book."
Includes index.
        1. Total hip replacement—Popular works.
        2. Total knee replacement—Popular works. I. Wolf, Eugene M. II. Title.
RD 549.S49   1999
617.5'810592—dc21
                                                                                98-44423
                                                                                CIP

ISBN 0-684-83920-2

Staring at that imposing word "Acknowledgments" in big letters up on my computer screen, I can't help but think of all the people who had something to do with bringing me to this moment. So many. Doctors, nurses, therapists, fellow patients, friends, family. And then I recall the first lines of John Donne's famous essay: "No man is an island, entire of itself; every man is a piece of the continent, a part of the main."

Suddenly I have one of those rare flashes when you know you've penetrated beyond the cliché and truly understand the words as though seeing them for the first time. And so, after three joint replacements, years of physical therapy, and the efforts of hundreds of others, I acknowledge what should always have been obvious: I am not an island—and how lucky I am that I'm not!

Of course, I'm not here thinking only of those who contributed directly to this book but to everyone who, one way or another, enabled me to enjoy the precious gift of a second life.

Therefore, I first want to thank all the scientific geniuses who devoted themselves to developing the concepts and the technology for knee and hip replacements. Without them I'd be sitting in a wheelchair. Their contribution to the human race stands on a par with the greatest achievements of the medical profession.

More particularly, I want to thank Dr. Eugene Wolf, my orthopedic surgeon, who not only gave me two new knees and a new hip but also gave me hope at a time when I was on the edge of despair. Dr. Wolf also encouraged me to put my story into a book that would help others in the same predicament. In addition to writing the Foreword to this book, Dr. Wolf participated in a series of taped interviews from which most of the basic medical information in this book is taken. And just to make sure I got it right, he reviewed the entire manuscript prior to publication.

Karen Sandy, my chief physical therapist, turned my belief that I would have a normal life again first into a conviction and then a practical enterprise. A veteran joint-replacement therapist, Karen has been associated with the Visiting Nurses Association of Northern California for a number of years. I can only wish that everyone getting a new knee or hip has someone like her to guide them through the rehabilitation process. Much of the information in these pages concerning physical therapy comes from Karen, who also reviewed the final manuscript.

Others in the medical and related professions who made valuable contributions to my physical well-being and/or this book include Dr. Susan Hoch, Associate Professor of Medicine at the Allegheny University of Health Sciences in Philadelphia, who also reviewed the manuscript and offered many useful suggestions; Dr. Stuart Zeman, of Oakland, whose arthroscopic surgeries on my knees bought me an additional four years before I had to turn to joint replacements; Craig Norton, the director of a sports medicine rehabilitation program at Alta-Bates Hospital in Oakland, who supervised my outpatient therapy and was of great help both in my rehab and with the sections on physical therapy; my good friend and neighbor Dr. Frank Anker, now retired, who gave me constant support and advice based both on his many years of experience as a physician and on his own total knee replacement.

Suzanne Graziano, Case Manager for the Arthoplasty Services Division of Nursing at the Hospital for Special Surgery in New York, was extremely helpful. Taking time from her busy schedule, Ms. Graziano escorted me through her facility, which specializes in joint-replacement surgery and other orthopedic treatments and is one of the finest of its kind in the United States. I particularly want to thank Ms. Graziano and the Hospital for Special Surgery for allowing me to use illustrations and portions of the text from its outstanding preop manuals for knee- and hip-replacement patients.

The Kaiser Permanente hospitals in Oakland and San Francisco allowed me to sit in on a preop class for hip-replacement patients and supplied me with copies of materials used in their patient education and physical therapy programs. The University of Iowa Hospitals and Clinics—another outstanding facility for joint replacements—likewise was generous in supplying patient education materials that proved useful in preparing the chapters dealing with that topic.

Frances Goldin and Sydelle Kramer of the Frances Goldin Literary Agency believed in the value of this project from the beginning and offered extremely useful suggestions on how to approach it. My editor, Bob Bender at Simon & Schuster, has been sensitive to the nuances of a book of this kind and has improved the original manuscript considerably.

One of the most gratifying aspects of writing this book is that it put me in touch—mostly via the Internet—with hundreds of my fellow joint-replacement patients. I have met only a few of them face to face, but I can say that they are among the most warmhearted souls I have ever encountered. They share the most personal experiences with people who are otherwise total strangers, and freely offer advice and support to one another at every turning point in our common journey. It was not possible to include all their stories and reflections in these pages, but I want to thank by name all those who shared their odysseys with me: Valerie Alia, Rose Marie Balan, Chris Barnsley, Ron Beddoe, Alexies Boulanov, Larry Burnam, Steve Colombo, Tim Dowd, Carol Downing, Ron Fowler, Walt Hanks, Brian Harris, Dietmar Hartl, Rob Hocker, Edna Jaffe, Elayne Jones, Bill Kennedy, John Kiefer, Maryanne Kufs, Gail Kuhn, Lady Andy, William Lalor, Mike Leggett, Harold Leventhal, Mairabet, Elizabeth "Betita" Martinez, Sally Pollock, Jane Schweitzer, Stacey Scott, Ann Sheehan, Edward Shineman, Jeff Solka, Ray Stewart, Doris Stokes, Joan Stuart, Roberta Suarez, Rebecca Wald, Donald Walden, Robert Walters, Anita Wilcox, Donald Wray.

My gratitude also to the gang at the Firehouse Tennis Court in Montclair, who, on my return to the tennis wars, made me feel right at home despite my obvious postop limitations. I can't mention all your names, but you know who you are. A special thanks, however, to two of you: Bill Bertetta, our court photographer, who documented via videotape the fact that I really do play tennis again and who supplied publicity photos to my publisher to be used in promoting this book; and the patron saint of the Firehouse Tennis Court, Jim Kenny, who, at the age of eighty-eight, continues to amaze everyone who knows him with his acerbic wisdom and his uncanny shotmaking.

Finally, thanks to my wife, Barbara Dane, who saw me through the worst of times and who continues to make the best of times even better.

For Barbara

CONTENTS

EUGENE M. WOLF, M.D.

I am an orthopedic surgeon at the California Pacific Medical Center in San Francisco, California. I operate on over four hundred patients every year for various injuries and diseases affecting their bones and joints.

Irwin Silber became one of those patients in 1993. He came to me because he had read an article in the *New York Times* about a technique I had developed for the transplantation of meniscal cartilage into damaged knees. As with many patients who hope to salvage their knees with a cartilage transplant, Irwin was not a proper candidate for this procedure. His knees were beyond cartilage transplantation. His only option was a total knee arthroplasty, an operative procedure that resurfaces the destroyed joint surfaces with metal and plastic components—generally known as a total knee replacement.

Although not the crux of my practice, joint-replacement surgery is a critically important process that I frequently use to restore arthritic patients to an active lifestyle. Over the next twelve months Irwin would undergo bilateral total knee arthroplasties and a left total hip arthroplasty.

When he came to my office in January 1993, he had previously been diagnosed as having painful and severely debilitating arthritis affecting both knees. The arthritis aside,

Irwin was a generally healthy sixty-seven-year-old gentle-man. But he could no longer walk comfortably for any distance or participate in a friendly game of doubles tennis. When I first saw him, Irwin was walking with a severe limp, using a cane. The arthritis not only precluded any sports activities, it also made the simple activities of daily living painful and grueling. The pain was present day and night, and kept him from sleeping comfortably.

Irwin's arthritis was of the degenerative type (osteoarthritis), the most common form; it is due to the wear and tear of the cartilage of our joints that our ever more active lives produce over time. There is no underlying destructive inflammatory disease process such as that found in rheumatoid arthritis or other inflammatory diseases, but it is a slowly progressive destruction of our primary weight-bearing joints that occurs for reasons that still remain obscure. It affects millions of Americans of all ages, although primarily in the older age groups; all races, and both sexes equally; and it leads to approximately 400,000 joint-replacement surgeries every year in the United States.

There are multiple reasons why someone is affected by degenerative arthritis, a term that includes different pathological entities with similar symptoms. The most common cause is the repetitive stresses of sports, work activities, and the activities of daily living. These will often produce arthritic changes in certain individuals who seem to have a propensity to develop arthritis. We are not all born with the same quality cartilage in our joints.

Why some individuals' joints can sustain repetitive stresses without noticeable wear or symptoms while other individuals seem to have less durable joints remains an enigma, although a family history of arthritis and joint replacement is common in persons who develop arthritis. One of the primary factors in the development of degenerative joint disease is trauma, and

Irwin had a history that is typical of patients with deteriorating joints due to injury.

Trauma occurs in different ways, but the most obvious type is a major episode that a person rarely forgets. It might occur in the course of a sporting event, in a motor vehicle accident, or with a simple wrong step and fall. In any case, the affected joint is immediately painful, swollen, and produces a significant functional limitation.

Irwin had such an episode in 1978. He fell while bicycling and landed on his right knee, which immediately became painful and swollen. His primary care physician, who treated him at that time, injected the knee with cortisone. No diagnostic tests were performed and MRI scans were not available then. Although he was improved by the cortisone injections, some significant cartilage damage probably occurred.

Could Irwin's knee have been restored to allow a normal lifestyle? In retrospect, it is difficult to say because treatment possibilities at that time were quite different from those of today, and the outcome might have been the same regardless of the best orthopedic care then available.

Orthopedic medicine has made dramatic progress over the last twenty years—progress I have been fortunate to witness and participate in as an orthopedic surgeon. We can now repair or reconstruct—and even regenerate—injured cartilage, ligaments, or bone in a damaged knee. New technologies have had an enormous impact on our present means of treatment in orthopedic surgery, and we can restore most patients to a normal, functional level.

Cartilage, ligament, or bone damage in any joint needs prompt attention by an orthopedic surgeon who, one hopes, can restore the joint to a normal anatomic situation. Only prompt restoration of the normal mechanics and structures will give a joint a chance of effectively serving its owner for the rest of his or her life. We can reconstruct that ligament or repair that cartilage, and the knee will appear to function normally, usually allowing a return to a normal lifestyle.

But I remind my patients that they were born with God-given structures, and I cannot match His work or preclude a recurrence of their injuries. And any joint that sustains significant trauma can go on to develop severe degenerative arthritis in subsequent years in spite of the best orthopedic care.

After his initial injury in 1978, Irwin was able to resume an active lifestyle, but he continued to have annoying symptoms during his tennis and other activities. At first he used the combination of Ben-Gay, aspirin, and an Ace bandage. As things worsened he resorted to anti-inflammatory medications, even tried physical therapy and dietary changes, but the arthritis worsened.

While on vacation in 1988, he experienced a bout of acute and severe pain in his right knee that led him to see his general practitioner, who referred him to a local orthopedic surgeon. Arthroscopic surgery was performed on the right knee in May 1989, and on the left knee in September 1990. Arthroscopic surgery is a minimally invasive procedure in which small tubes are inserted into a joint to allow us to remove any loose or frayed cartilage.

These arthroscopic procedures helped Irwin for about two to three years, but then the pain and swelling came back stronger than ever. The orthopedic surgeon who had performed the arthroscopies then told Irwin he needed a total knee arthroplasty. Seeking other options, Irwin next went to a rheumatologist—a medical doctor who specializes in the nonoperative or medical treatment of arthritis. The rheumatologist recommended a course of treatment based on the prescription of prednisone, a cortisone derivative. Mr. Silber declined this recommendation and next sought treatment from a homeopathic doctor, who prescribed multiple herbs and pills. Irwin tried these, but they had no significant effect.

After having explored all the possible options available for the treatment of his arthritis, Mr. Silber limped bravely into my office on January 26, 1993. On his initial visit it was evident that all conservative and nonoperative means of treatment had been exhausted. His functional limitations were obvious, and the pain was apparent on his face.

At age sixty-seven, and considering the level of destruction his knees had sustained, it was clear that a cartilage transplant was out of the question. The only decision to be made at that time was whether to go ahead with a total knee arthroplasty or a less-invasive procedure, a unicompartmental arthroplasty. As opposed to a total knee arthroplasty that resurfaces all of the articular surfaces of the knee, a unicompartmental arthroplasty resurfaces only part of the knee. The recovery following unicompartmental arthroplasty is much easier, and the functional result obtained is superior, but it can be performed in patients who have only one compartment of the knee predominantly affected.

I then performed an in-office diagnostic arthroscopy under local anesthesia to determine whether a unicompartmental arthroplasty was a possibility. Diagnostic arthroscopy is the most accurate standard for determining the presence or absence of intra-articular pathology.

As it turned out, the arthroscopy of Irwin's right knee showed that the entire joint was severely affected and a total knee arthroplasty was the only option. On March 15, 1993, the right total knee arthroplasty was performed. After a successful right knee surgery we repeated the procedure on the left knee on November 8, 1993, and then did the left hip on March 14, 1994.

Less than a year after his operations, Irwin was not only

back to a normal existence with respect to routine activities of daily living, he was also winning games on the tennis court.

I next saw Irwin early in 1997, when he told me that he had decided to write a book about his experience. After twenty years of orthopedic practice, this was a first for me. Although I knew Mr. Silber was an accomplished and well-published writer, I asked myself why anyone would be interested in a book about his total joint experience.

But on further discussion of Mr. Silber's concept of his book, I realized that his goal—providing prospective joint-replacement patients with better and more extensive information on the entire procedure from a patient's point of view—was indeed a most useful undertaking.

Orthopedic surgeons are focused on their ability to take someone who is suffering from an injured or arthritic joint and is unable to enjoy an active lifestyle, and return that person to a new and higher level of activity. In that pursuit we are concerned with identifying the disease processes and determining the proper course of treatment. When the disease process has led to the destruction of a knee or hip joint, the solution is often a joint replacement, or what we call a total joint arthroplasty.

The destructive arthritic processes can produce severe bony deformities that often pose technical obstacles to the successful performance of a total joint arthroplasty. Your orthopedic surgeon's main goal in total joint replacement is to overcome those obstacles and provide you with a knee or hip that is technically perfect, so that you can enjoy a lifetime of pain-free activity. If the performance of the surgery is compromised in any way, the viability of the prosthesis that has been inserted will be shortened. We are obsessed with the pursuit of surgical perfection and with the careful postoperative care needed to avoid the major complications that may arise from such surgery.

That continuous pursuit does not allow us as individual surgeons to adequately prepare and educate patients about what they will experience. Patients need to know as much as possible about the entire process from the moment they check into the hospital to the completion of their physical therapy program.

Having reviewed Mr. Silber's book while it was still in manuscript form, I am certain that the information provided here will go a long way toward providing the knowledge necessary to allay most of the fears that arise when someone is faced with the prospect of a total joint operation. Hospitals are assuming a larger role in that education process, but this book provides invaluable detail and information to prepare a patient for the total joint experience.

In 1997 orthopedic surgeons in the United States performed almost 400,000 total knee and hip replacements. That number is growing each year.

As a result of this relatively new medical technology, many people who thought they were fated to spend the rest of their days in a wheelchair or walking in pain—and even then only with the help of a cane or a walker—have resumed normal lives.

I am one of those people.

You might even say that, statistically speaking, I'm three of them, since during one twelve-month period, from March 1993 to March 1994, I had three total joint replacements—both knees and my left hip. Today I walk without a cane, ride a bike, play tennis and, in general, lead a normal life.

How did that happen and what was the experience like? That's what this book is about.

This book is not about arthritis, although arthritis is the principal cause of the pain and disability that lead many people to consider joint replacement. Nor is this a book that will tell you how to adjust your life to the crippling effects of arthritis. There are many other books that do that.

Rather, this is a book about the most revolutionary new development for the treatment of the consequences of the most severe cases of arthritis in the past hundred years: the replacement of crippled and diseased joints—most particularly hips and knees—with artificial prostheses. This procedure has already enabled hundreds of thousands of people to regain a quality of life they thought had been lost forever.

As the title says, this is a *patient's* guide to knee and hip replacements. It is written not from a doctor's perspective but a patient's, by someone who has gone through the experience not once but three times. The idea for writing this book first came to me when I was told that I needed what turned out to be a series of joint replacements. But when I asked my orthopedic surgeon to suggest a book on the subject that I could read, he told me that aside from technical books written for the medical community, there weren't any.

It wasn't until much later—after I had my new joints—that I realized just how helpful such a book would have been for me. And so, in this book, I have tried to reproduce as much of my experience as I thought would be relevant for others facing the prospect of joint-replacement surgery: what I went through when my arthritis first became symptomatic; the buying-time measures various doctors recommended; why joint replacements were finally recommended; how I found an orthopedic surgeon in whom I felt confident; the factors that went into my decision; the scores of questions I had going in, only some of which were answered in my preop discussions with my surgeon; my anxieties about the surgery; the operation itself; and, not least, the rehabilitation process.

Although I am not a doctor, many of the medical aspects of joint replacements are also discussed. That information is based on a series of lengthy interviews with my orthopedic surgeon, Dr. Eugene Wolf, the most active orthopedic surgeon at the California-Pacific Medical Center in San Francisco. I have digested this information into what I hope readers will find is readily accessible language. Dr. Wolf has also reviewed the final manuscript to make sure that my interpretation of medical language is substantively accurate.

.   .   .

In 1989, after experiencing increasing pain in my right knee, I was diagnosed as having extensive arthritis in both my knees and my hips. Various treatments—special exercises, physical therapy, cortisone shots, other painkillers, and arthroscopic surgery—provided temporary relief. But after a while, they were no longer effective. The pain returned even more strongly than before. When it did, it became more difficult for me to pursue normal activities. Meanwhile, I had become totally dependent on nonsteroidal anti-inflammatory drugs (NSAIDs) just to get by each day.

I was sixty-three years old at the time and had worked all my life as a journalist. In my later years, especially, my work often brought me to parts of the world where the facilities posed real challenges to anyone with a handicap. (I had been to Vietnam, Cambodia, China, Cuba, the USSR, and many other places where hotel accommodations and means of transportation were often an adventure in themselves.) When I wasn't working, I played tennis four or five times a week. (People who know about such things rated me a "High B.") I went bike riding, swam, hiked, and walked extensively. I also did much of the cooking and shopping at home.

But as my condition worsened, my activity was severely curtailed. More and more my work was at my desk. My last trip abroad was to the (former) Soviet Union in 1989. (With my leg elevated on a pillow, I watched the fall of the Berlin Wall on Soviet television from my hotel room in Moscow.) Over the next few years I worked on a book that explored the historical and theoretical sources of the Soviet collapse. But as the book neared completion, even sitting at my computer was getting uncomfortable. The last few months before I finished it in the fall of 1993 became a race against time. (The book, *Socialism: What Went Wrong?* was published a year later.)

Tennis, of course, was out of the question. Any weight-bearing activity, including walking, was extremely painful. Driving was getting more and more difficult. My contributions to my family's daily living needs became memories. Increasingly, I found myself sitting in my recliner, avoiding the moment of ambulation. (The inanity of most television programming turned out to be my friend. Without it I might be sitting in that chair still.)

Nature's calls were a constant source of trepidation until a friend suggested I get a raised toilet seat. But although that somewhat solved the physical problem, it was an ongoing reminder that I faced a future laced with increasing indignities. The pain even went to bed with me at night.

By then my life had begun to revolve around my arthritis. I was living on powerful antipain drugs—not just NSAIDs but even more powerful painkillers such as Vicodin. And the prospect facing me was that my condition would only get worse. I had dismal visions of myself housebound, if not wheelchair-bound, for the rest of my life. Years later I was in touch—via the Internet—with a fellow sufferer who captured my feelings perfectly. "I hate the thought," he wrote, "that the disease defines who I am."

Eventually, the time I had bought with three rounds of arthroscopic surgery on my knees ran out, and I became convinced that my only alternative was total joint replacement. So during one twelve-month period starting in March 1993 I had both knees and my left hip replaced. The surgery was performed by Dr. Eugene Wolf at the California-Pacific Medical Center in San Francisco.

That stretch was one of the most difficult I've ever been through. I felt as though my life had become one long surgery. While recovering from one operation I was preparing for the next. I couldn't tell where the pain from the surgery left off and the pain from the next area of distress began. A month before the last of my joint replacements (my hip, in March 1994), the pain had become so unbearable that I was counting the days and then the hours until I would once again be lying on the operating table waiting to hear the anesthesiologist say those increasingly familiar words: "Sweet dreams!"

Nevertheless, it was also a period of great optimism. Starting the day after my first knee replacement, I felt that I was on the road to reclaiming the rest of my life. Physical therapy was not only a means of regaining the use of my joints, it was a way of taking control of my rehabilitation. Two months after the last operation, I was able to do a daily one-mile walk by myself. Four months later, carried away by my progress, I ventured out to the wall adjacent to my favorite tennis court to see what I could do. Actually, not much. It would be another six months before I'd try again.

But in October 1994, when my book came out, just seven months after my hip was replaced, I went on a one-month speaking tour across the country promoting my book and telling audiences what I thought had gone wrong with the Soviet attempt to construct a socialist system. (If you're interested in my opinions on that subject, you'll have to read the book.)

Now I'm in my mid-seventies and I lead a relatively normal life. I do not use a cane or a walker. I drive, can walk several miles at a stretch, and, much to my family's relief—at least that's what they say—I am back to cooking. I am also taking out the garbage, changing lightbulbs, cleaning out the cats' litter box, and undertaking similarly challenging chores with equanimity. And, much to everyone's surprise, including my own, I am playing tennis again—mostly doubles but even an occasional set of singles. I am also riding my bike and navigating stairs and even (not unduly steep) hills. My wife can take extended trips without fear of leaving me alone. (And the raised toilet seat is on a shelf in my closet.)

No, I can't do everything. Certain activities, like gardening, that require constant stooping and bending are too uncomfortable. I don't carry anything weighing more than twenty pounds. I shouldn't go up a ladder or sit down on the floor—getting down from the former and up from the latter are difficult—but I've done both in an emergency. I avoid low chairs and couches, and I feel a lot more secure if there's a banister when I go up and down stairs.

Although I live with the likelihood that sooner or later my other hip will probably also have to be replaced, my doctor and my physical therapist consider me a "success story." (Since I can cover almost as much court as many others in my ever-skeptical geriatric tennis crowd, they are not convinced that I actually have had three joints replaced.) In fact, my wife and I are so optimistic that we sold our single-level, elevator-accessible condominium and bought a split-level house.

Now hardly a week passes without my getting a call from a prospective knee- or hip-replacement candidate who wants to talk to someone who has been there and done that. And that's why I've written this book.

Obviously, no book can answer specific medical questions about your condition and whether or not you are a likely candidate for a joint replacement. Only your doctor can do that. Nor should my experience be taken as an exact model for anyone else's treatment. Although there are no known "cures" for arthritis, there are various treatments for it, depending on its stage of development. In fact, a joint replacement is usually the last resort, used only when the disease is so far advanced that the alternatives no longer help. There are also many variations in joint-replacement surgery depending on the source of the patient's ailment, his or her physical condition and age, new developments in the field, and the orthopedic surgeon's particular methodology. (Keep in mind, too, that since this book is based principally on my own experience, its focus is on knee and hip replacements. Not coincidentally, these are the most common joint replacements.)

On the other hand, my experience is far from unique. That became clear after interviews with my orthopedic surgeon and my physical therapists and by talking (directly and on the Internet) to scores of people who have had knee and/or hip replacements. Most have been successful. A few have not. And although no two patients (or surgeons, for that matter) are exactly alike, the basic elements of the procedure are pretty much the same.

This book is designed to do two things:

1. Enable the reader to get a vivid idea of what's involved in a joint replacement from a patient's point of view by seeing and feeling it through my experience.

2. Help the reader more fully understand the key elements in this experience, including the various options available at each stage of the process; alternatives to joint-replacement surgery; what to expect in the preop period; what the surgeon actually does in the operating room; the recovery process; managing with your new knee or hip; the role and different stages of physical therapy; the risks involved in this type of surgery; and what the patient can reasonably expect in the long term.

I hope that by enabling you to share an experience you might currently be contemplating, this book will help demystify the entire process and not only help you get through your surgery—if that's the course you opt for—but also help you get the best possible results from it.

Good luck!

CHAPTER 1

Life Before the Knife

A "Touch" of Arthritis

Five years before my first total knee replacement, when I was sixty-four years old, my doctor told me that the progressively worsening pain in my right knee was from arthritis. The news was not exactly a surprise. Like many others, my first reaction was to shrug it off. After all, didn't most people my age get what's casually referred to as a "touch" of arthritis? Besides, although that knee had been bothering me for more than twelve years—the result of an unfortunate encounter between my bike and a New York City pothole—it had not significantly altered my daily life.

I didn't know it at the time, of course, but—as is frequently the case—that accident was probably what triggered the onset of my arthritis in my right knee. (Although there is evidence of a genetic component to arthritis, neither of my parents had any visible signs of the disease. In fact, my father lived to be ninety, and until he developed Alzheimer's at the age of eighty-seven, would regularly walk three to four miles a day.)

Unlike previous injuries, however, my pothole mishap produced problems that never completely cleared up. Physical therapy and occasional cortisone shots eased the pain, but sooner or later the pain would come back with increasing intensity. Still, I was able to lead a reasonably normal life for the next ten years. The main visible difference was the variety of Ace bandages I put on my knees when engaging in any kind of physical activity. Increasingly, the aroma of Ben-Gay pungently announced my presence on the tennis court. (Years later, my orthopedist told me that mainly the bandage probably helped me psychologically, functioning as a reminder that my right knee should not be overburdened.

In time, the pain in my right knee began to be duplicated in the left—a development I attributed to the extra load my left knee was probably carrying. At the same time, the pain came more frequently and was gradually getting stronger. What I didn't realize was that an irreversible arthritic process had begun and the disease was in the process of softening, tearing, and eroding the cartilage in my major weight-bearing joints. It was most advanced in my knees—probably because, having by then moved to California, I was playing even more tennis than I did back east.

As the pain intensified, it was clear that this time things would be different—although I still didn't know how different. It was then that X rays revealed that I had what the American Academy of Orthopedic Surgeons (AAOS) calls "the most common cause of chronic knee pain and disability"—osteoarthritis.

Although I was also beginning to have similar symptoms in my hips, my knees were the most affected. This is the most common pattern in the development of osteoarthritis as shown by the fact that there are more total knee arthroplasties (that's the medical term for joint replacements) than any other type. But I wasn't ready for new joints yet.

Learning About Arthritis

Like most people, I had always thought of arthritis as a disease of old age, and to me—as for most of us—old age was something that was always going to happen later on. In a way, aside from the pain, that's the most daunting aspect of finding out that you have arthritis. It's an ungracious signal that "later on" has arrived. At least it was for me.

After learning that I had arthritis—I didn't even know enough then to ask what type I had—the first thing I wanted to know was how to get rid of it. "Which do you want first," asked my doctor, "the good news or the bad news?"

Figuring it's always better to go out on a positive note, I asked for the bad news first. He went straight to the point: "There is no cure!"

After that I wasn't sure how good the good news could be, but it was somewhat encouraging. First, he told me I had osteoarthritis, which, he explained, was not as debilitating to the body as a whole as other forms, such as rheumatoid arthritis. Second, osteoarthritis is not a life-threatening disease. And third, there are treatments that can ease the pain, increase mobility, and in some cases, even slow down the progress of the disease.

So I decided I'd read up on arthritis. I got hold of some literature from the Arthritis Foundation. (There's a branch in most major cities, or you can write to them at P.O. Box 19000, Atlanta, GA 30326.) I found books on arthritis in the public library. I checked out various newsletters dealing with health issues—*Consumer Reports, Mayo Clinic,* the *UC Berkeley Wellness Letter,* the *Harvard Health Letter,* and so on—and found that they frequently carried articles on arthritis and arthritis treatments. I suddenly became aware of the numerous newspaper and magazine articles dealing with arthritis, and friends began sending me pieces I might otherwise have missed. I also found some news groups on the Internet: alt.support.arthritis and misc.health.arthritis.

Most of what I read repeated and amplified what my doctor had told me: The disease is treatable but there is no cure.

Osteoarthritis

One of the first things I learned when I set out to know more about my condition was that there are different forms of arthritis and that while some symptoms are common to most, many are distinct diseases requiring specific treatments.

The most common is osteoarthritis, which has been called "man's oldest and most common disease." That's what I have. Osteoarthritis tends to strike later in life, although it can attack at any age.

According to James Gamble of the Division of Orthopaedic Surgery at the Stanford University School of Medicine, "Eighty-five percent of people between the ages of 70 and 79 have radiographically observable osteoarthritis, and 80 percent of those over 55 have clinical evidence of osteoarthritis in at least one joint (most commonly the knee)."[*]

---

[*]*The Musculoskeletal System* (New York: Raven Press, 1988).

Since osteoarthritis mostly affects people forty-five and older, it is generally assumed that the wear and tear of daily living is a significant factor in the disease.

The next most common form is secondary to an injury. This is very similar to osteoarthritis and is known as post-traumatic arthritis.

No one knows for sure how many people have underlying quiescent arthritic changes, since many years can pass before the disease becomes symptomatic. Estimates range anywhere from 16 to 45 million people in the United States alone. But according to Dr. William Reynolds, Director of Medical and Scientific Affairs for the U.S. Arthritis Foundation, its incidence is even more widespread. "It is certain," says Reynolds, "that every person over 60 could be found to have it to some degree." Fortunately, he adds, "only a small percentage of those with osteoarthritis have it badly enough to notice it."

Unfortunately, mine is the noticeable kind.

Osteoarthritis is not difficult to diagnose, but there is no single, clearly defined cause or offending agent such as a virus or bacteria. Heredity, lifestyle, overuse, and/or abuse of the joint certainly play a role in its development. Doctors have a tremendous amount of information about the pathological process—the physiology of what happens to the chemical properties of cartilage and bone in osteoarthritis. But that's still a far cry from understanding this chronic destructive process, let alone reversing it.

Many alternative practitioners believe that osteoarthritis stems from a breakdown in the body's autoimmune system due to an inadequate supply of certain nutrients or enzymes.

There is little doubt, however, about what the disease does. The characteristic feature of osteoarthritis is the progressive weakening and degeneration of the articular cartilage in the affected joint.* As the cartilage gradually erodes and the increasingly cushionless articular surfaces rub against each other, you experience increasing stiffness, inflammation, swelling, pain, lack of mobility, and bone deformity.

Its favorite targets are the hands (where it shows up especially in the fingers), the knees, the hips, and the spine. Most doctors can diagnose osteoarthritis from a physical examination, but X rays are an important means of verifying the diagnosis. An X ray doesn't "see" cartilage, so a normal joint will show a space where the cartilage separates and covers the bony surfaces. As the cartilage gets destroyed, that space disappears and the bone begins to react and change shape. Eventually, if the cartilage is totally eroded, the raw, bony surfaces will rub against each other, causing even greater pain and deformity.

Since osteoarthritis develops slowly and usually becomes symptomatic later in life, it does not significantly impinge on most people's ability to function more or less normally during the early phases of the disease. In many cases, antipain medicines—NSAIDs, occasional cortisone shots, exercise, and diet changes, for example—can reduce pain sufficiently so that you can go on with your life while making minor adjustments. In more advanced cases, there is an accumulation of debris from the weakened and/or torn cartilage. Surrounding tissues become inflamed, causing even more intense pain and limited mobility. A relatively minor procedure, arthroscopic surgery, can clean out the joint and enable the person to function more or less normally—at least for a while. But the level of relief obtained by arthroscopic surgery can vary greatly depending on the level of joint destruction and deformity and the severity of the disease.

It is only when these measures no longer provide signifi-

---

*Articular cartilage is the particular type of cartilage in the joints, as distinguished from other types of cartilage in the body.

cant relief from the pain, stiffness, and increasing lack of mobility that more drastic actions may be called for.

The idea of surgically replacing a severely damaged joint with an artificial joint goes back at least to the late part of the nineteenth century, when an ivory hip was fashioned and cemented into place . Later on, glass and Teflon were tried, but it was not until the introduction of new metal alloys and polyethylene in the 1960s that these efforts were successful.

Fortunately for me, the two most successful procedures were knee and hip replacements. Since their inception, the surgical techniques and the prostheses have improved many times over so that today these surgeries have a success rate of more than 95 percent. Knee and hip replacements account for more than 80 percent of all joint replacements, totaling between them more than 300,000 a year in the United States alone. Other joint-replacement operations are for the shoulder, elbow, wrist, and small joints of the hand.

Rheumatoid Arthritis

Rheumatoid arthritis, which is a less widespread but more debilitating disease, usually begins earlier—between the ages of twenty-one and forty-five—and affects roughly 2.5 million Americans. For some reason, its incidence among women is three times that in men. It is also a systemic disease; that is, it affects the whole body, not just the joints. The Arthritis Foundation calls it "the most dangerous, destructive and disabling" of all forms of arthritis.

Generally considered an autoimmune disease—that is, one in which the body attacks itself and begins destroying its own cells and tissues—rheumatoid arthritis usually starts with inflammation of the connective tissue (synovial lining) of a joint, and then destroys the entire joint.

"The most obvious damage," says the *Harvard Health Letter Special Report on Arthritis*, "occurs in joints, but the disease affects the whole body. Inflammation may harm the heart, lungs, blood vessels, eyes, lymph lodes or spleen. The body's ongoing battle with inflammation is exhausting and can cause fatigue, fever, weakness, loss of appetite and weight, and anemia."

"In about one [case] in six," the FDA reports, "the disease becomes severe and can shorten life."

One notable difference between osteoarthritis and rheumatoid arthritis is that osteoarthritis patients usually don't feel sick. Even when my pain was getting unbearable, I remember having the sense that—except for the arthritis—I was healthy.

Rheumatoid arthritis is also frequently the source of devastating and near-constant pain. "Can anyone tell me how you explain to someone who doesn't have rheumatoid arthritis what it feels like?" writes Larry Burnam in Pleasanton, Texas. "I am no longer able to work in my chosen profession as a heavy equipment mechanic. I have worked at odd jobs from February 1992 when I was diagnosed with rheumatoid arthritis until October 1996 when I had to quit altogether. I can't quite find a strong enough term to make anyone understand. Sometimes I tell them that it's like a total body tooth ache, but even that doesn't really hit the mark."

Although there are many differences between osteoarthritis and rheumatoid arthritis—in origin, course of development, and so forth—both wind up attacking, weakening, and destroying articular cartilage. Consequently, you may get to the point where a joint replacement becomes an attractive option no matter which form of arthritis you have.

Joint replacements can benefit both patients with rheumatoid arthritis (RA) and patients with osteoarthritis (OA). Since their general physical condition is usually better, OA patients' joint replacements generally require less technically demanding surgery. RA patients often have a more painful and destructive disease, greater deformity, and weaker bones (often as a consequence of the high use of cortisone needed to control their disease). But their pain relief after a joint replacement can be even more dramatic. They may also have problems using crutches or a walker because of inflammation in finger, wrist, or elbow joints. On the other hand, the lower activity level of RA patients produces less wear on their prostheses.

It's also possible to have aspects of both osteoarthritis and rheumatoid arthritis or a combination of any of the different types of arthritis.

These are the two main types of arthritis. Other common types are gout, psoriatic arthritis, juvenile arthritis, ankylosing spondylitis,* and systemic lupus erythematosus. Joint replacements can often help people with these forms of arthritis as well.

Exercise

None of this is to say that you're doomed to a life of increasing pain and physical confinement if you have arthritis. After all, most people with arthritis— especially osteoarthritis—never get to the point of needing a joint replacement. But even if, like me, you turn out to be in that sizable minority who can no longer tough it out on their own, there are treatments that can ease the pain,

---

* The American Medical Association describes ankylosing spondylitis as an "inflammation of the joints that link the vertebrae. . . . [When] the inflammation recedes [it] leaves behind hardened, damaged joints that effectively fuse together the separate bones of the spinal column."

increase mobility, and, in some cases, even slow down the progress of the disease. These are not small achievements. Osteoarthritis tends to be a slow-developing disease, so the alleviation of its main symptoms can, by itself, make it possible for most people with this most common form of the affliction to lead relatively normal lives.

Perhaps the single most important thing someone with arthritis can do is exercise. And not just once in a while. Of course, this is easier said than done. Many people who develop arthritis late in life have been relatively sedentary, and suddenly—just when they're feeling the aches and pains—they're being advised to start exercising. Even for those who have always been active in sports, such advice might come off as gratuitous. That's the way I felt as my arthritis became an increasingly significant factor in determining what I could and couldn't do.

For thirty-five years, my favorite physical activity was tennis. So—wouldn't you know it?—of all the things I liked to do, tennis was the hardest to keep up. Gradually I found myself cutting back. First I found that I just didn't feel like playing two days in a row. Then I found that I was looking for older partners. (My usual practice had been singles with players half my age.) Then it was doubles rather than singles.

Eventually I had to stop. That was one of the low points in my arthritis odyssey. So I started thinking about possible alternatives and came up with two: swimming and bike riding.

My hunches were backed up by the doctors. Swimming, especially, is considered by many experts the ideal exercise for those with arthritis. It's a nonimpact, non-weight-bearing aerobic exercise that not only can strengthen muscles around your joints but also provides excellent cardiovascular conditioning.

I was particularly fortunate in finding a pool that was tailor-made for my needs. Only a five-minute drive from my house, the Dimond Park Lions Pool (donated to the people of Oakland by the Lions Club) is an all-year, outdoor, lifeguard-attended, heated pool with a five-day-a-week senior swim at a cost of $1.25 per session. It also has water exercise classes, which are especially helpful for non-swimmers.

I went faithfully three times a week, but my swimming form leaves a lot to be desired. I don't use my legs enough. I think that's true of most casual swimmers. So I devised some ways of exercising my legs more. First, I swam with flippers, which gave my knees more resistance in the water. (It was also more fun.) This enabled me to swim on my back, propelling myself along only with a continuous kicking motion. I would do this every third lap. Finally, I would stand in one corner of the shallow end (4.5 feet) of the pool and, resting my arms on the pool wall, kick up and down with each leg—a set of ten kicks ten times.

The biggest drawback to swimming—at least for me—was that it was boring. So I had to keep reminding myself how good it was for me. And it was. Swimming regularly, I was able to measure my gains quickly. My first day, I managed two laps (four lengths of thirty-five yards each) and found myself out of breath—despite all my years of tennis. But after four months, I was routinely swimming a minimum of a half mile (thirteen laps) every time out. After a while, my breathing got stronger and my pulse rate settled into a healthy sixty beats per minute.

Senior swim was also a social occasion. Most of the swimmers were regulars and we all had a litany of conditions to share with each other. There were, of course, others with arthritis as well as people who'd had bypass surgery or strokes, and some with just plain getting-old aches and pains. And there were those who just loved to swim. One eighty-five-year-old woman regularly participated in the Senior Olympics and had medals to show for it.

Sure, I'm lucky to have the Lions Pool almost in my back-yard and to live in the San Francisco Bay Area, where it's pos-sible to swim outdoors in a heated pool all year-round. But equivalent facilities can be found almost everywhere. (Inci-dentally, many Y's offer financial assistance to people who can't afford their membership fees. Just ask.)

Also, keep in mind that there's a lot more to water exercises than swimming. Some require special classes. Many can be done on your own. Most local chapters of the Arthritis Foundation offer a specially devised program of arthritis aquatics. These are usually held in facilities where the fees are nominal and the con-ditions are suited to the needs of people with arthritis.

Bike riding is another good aerobic, non-weight-bearing activity, but it should be approached with care. For me, it wasn't so much a matter of getting into it as continuing it. I'm not a big-time cyclist, but my wife and I had ridden our bikes regularly about once a week when we were living in Brooklyn, and we continued to do so when we moved to Cal-ifornia. But as my arthritis developed—and as we both got older—neither of us felt quite as secure breezing through traf-fic as we used to. So, I got a bike rack for my car and we found several traffic-free, mostly flat bike paths, and that became a regular part of my exercise regimen.

Cycling might be one of the few exercises you can do even when you're in a lot of pain. Tim Dowd has ankylosing spondylitis, an inflammatory arthritis that primarily attacks the spine and sometimes the hips and shoulders. "I let the pain and discouragement of the disease turn me into a couch potato for too many years," Tim writes, "and paid a great price for it. Finally, through a process of trial and error, I dis-covered cycling. It's joint-friendly, very aerobic and a lot of fun. Regular riding has definitely improved my quality of life, reduced the amount of pain I experience and improved my self-esteem. Getting a good workout helps reduce the current pain I feel most of the time."

Aside from sports like swimming and bike riding, there are many exercise programs specifically designed to help people with arthritis. Your doctor might be able to give you some advice and, even better, recommend a physical therapist. The Arthritis Foundation (call 800-283-7800 to locate your local chapter) gives exercise classes it calls PACE (People with Arthritis Can Exercise) and also provides an exercise videotape.

You'll find a shelf full of books dealing with arthritis at your local library or in major bookstores such as Borders and Barnes and Noble. Many of these have extensive illustrated sections filled with useful tips on exercises you can do at home, stretching and strengthening exercises, aerobic exercises, and aquatic exercises. Two that I have found useful are *Arthritis Relief,* by Jean Wallace (Rodale Press), and *The Arthritis Helpbook,* by Kate Lorig (a doctor of physical therapy) and Dr. James Fries (Addison-Wesley).

You might also look into tai chi, the Chinese slow-motion dancelike movements based on the relaxation of the large muscles, flexibility of the joints, deep breathing, and balanced body movements.

Then there are lots of things that are just plain common sense. For instance, if you're overweight, take off some pounds. This will reduce the strain on your weight-bearing joints. And avoid high-impact and body-twisting sports such as football, jogging, hockey, volleyball, and racquetball—all of which will exacerbate your pain. Also, consider any task-related motions that might be unduly stressful on your joints. Use a cane or crutches to help you walk while reducing the pressure on your joints. (Either one will do wonders for getting you a seat on a crowded bus or train.)

Medications

There are medications that have proven effective in combating pain and improving mobility. Perhaps the most widely used is one or another of the numerous nonsteroidal anti-inflammatory drugs (NSAIDs). These come in both prescription and over-the-counter strength. Aspirin and ibuprofen are among those you can get without a prescription. Unfortunately, as with so many other things in life, the use of such medications is a trade-off. All have side effects that, over time, can provoke discomfort in the gastrointestinal tract and in some cases have led to ulcers. But they do provide relief. Tylenol is also good for pain, but it is not an anti-inflammatory. And although it doesn't lead to gastrointestinal problems, long-term use might cause damage in the liver and/or kidneys.

Like most people, I felt that the risks were worth the benefit. I wouldn't want to be dependent on NSAIDs for the rest of my life, and I keep hoping that someone will come up with one that's free of negative side effects. You might want to start with an over-the-counter NSAID to see what it does for you. Ibuprofen—the generic name for more expensive name brands such as Advil—has worked well for me.

If you need something stronger, ask your doctor for a recommendation. For one thing, these drugs are pretty expensive. Since doctors usually get free samples, you can see which you can tolerate before making a big investment in one. After trying several, I settled on Feldene, one of the most powerful. My digestive tract seemed able to handle it for a while, but when I began to feel some discomfort in my stomach, I switched to Lodine. There are also reports of a new type of NSAID that supposedly does not produce negative side effects.

Dr. Susan Hoch, a rheumatologist and an associate professor of medicine at Allegheny University of Health Sciences in Philadelphia, notes: "There are some milder anti-inflammatories you might consider, including Trilisate or Salflex. In my experience, Dolobid is another relatively less toxic NSAID, as is Lodine. Regardless of which one you choose, I would only take it along with Cytotec (200 mg qid), which protects the stomach lining by maintaining the gastric barrier to acid."

Don't be surprised if by the time you read this there is a new batch of NSAIDs available that are less irritating to the stomach. One such is Arthrotec, which, according to a review in the *European Journal of Rheumatology and Inflammation,* "provides powerful anti-inflammatory efficacy with enhanced upper GI safety." Other medications are currently in clinical trial.

This is an area where alternative medicine might prove its worth. I'd be a bit leery about completely trashing medications that clearly provide relief in favor of a remedy—or a combination of remedies—that might take months to kick in. But if you're open to the idea, you might want to experiment with reducing your intake of NSAIDs while starting on some food supplements—vitamins, enzymes, and Chinese herbs, for example—as prescribed by a reputable alternative practitioner.

Glucosamine and Chondroitin Sulfates and "The Arthritis Cure"

You might also look into glucosamine and chondroitin sulfates, the "natural" medications recommended by Dr. Jason Theodosakis in his recent book, *The Arthritis Cure.* Because the book's title and promotional material are good examples of overhype, many professionals have been understandably dubious about them.

The promise of an "arthritis cure" would be astounding. But the book begins with an "Important Note to Readers" that states: "We use the word *cure* to mean the partial or complete relief of symptoms. . . . Nothing in the title or content of this book is intended to suggest that the use of the recommended supplements will fully eradicate osteoarthritis."

In fact, the claims actually made in the book are somewhat more modest.

Theodosakis cites numerous veterinarians who have used glucosamine and chondroitin sulfates on animals with significantly positive results. He also cites cases in which glucosamine and chondroitin sulfates have been taken by people who report a marked lessening of pain without the side effects often experienced with the usual medications. What might be of even greater significance in the long run is Theodosakis's claim that glucosamine and chondroitin sulfates provide "a simple, safe and effective means of encouraging cartilage repair."

The good news about glucosamine and/or the combination of glucosamine and chondroitin sulfates is that a number of people who have tried them report that these medications relieve pain and stiffness in the joints. Also, several clinical studies suggest, in the words of one, that "oral glucosamine sulfate is as effective as a standard NSAID such as ibuprofen in controlling the symptoms of [osteoarthritis] with clinically evident signs of inflammation, while it is significantly better tolerated."*

Dr. Hoch believes that what's needed is for some institu-

*L. C. Rovati, "Clinical Research in Osteoarthritis: Design and Results of Short-Term and Long-Term Trials with Disease-Modifying Drugs," *International Journal of Tissue Reactions* (1992). Dr. Rovati is affiliated with the Department of Clinical Pharmacology, Roota Research Laboratory, Monza, Italy.

tion "such as the Section of Alternative Medicine of the National Institutes of Health to fund a long-term study [of glucosamine and chondroitin sulfates] looking at such things as joint fluid, x-rays over time, etc. rather than just pain which can be a placebo effect in a believer."

Although it might turn out that glucosamine and chondroitin sulfates will add another tool to the growing body of treatments for arthritis, it is certainly far too soon to claim that the oral ingestion of glucosamine sulfate can repair or regenerate cartilage. That would take far more elaborate clinical studies over a significant period of time to determine.

But even if glucosamine and chondroitin sulfates do no more than provide a side effect–free possible alternative to aspirin, NSAIDs, and cortisone, it will be a major improvement on some of the most widely used current medical treatments. However, it can hardly be considered a cure.

Diet

A change in diet might also help. For a long time, most doctors scoffed at the idea that there might be a connection between diet and arthritis. Even as the medical profession acknowledged that foods high in fat and cholesterol probably play a role in the development of heart disease and cancer, resistance to linking diet to arthritis continued. Fortunately, this attitude is beginning to change. Today, everyone suggests following a diet low in red meat and other high-cholesterol foods, eating more fruit and vegetables, and making sure you're getting a good intake of fiber. It's probably also a good idea to reduce your intake of alcohol (sorry about that!), salt, and sugar.

Perhaps if you start early enough, this kind of diet can help reduce the chances of your developing arthritis. Unfortunately, by the time arthritis symptoms are noticeable, the disease has usually advanced beyond the point where diet can reverse it. But the diet will be good for you anyway and, at the very least, will strengthen your body as it copes with arthritis. And it might actually slow down the progress of the disease.

I don't know if, in my case, cause and effect were at work. But at the time of my hip replacement, Dr. Wolf thought I might be going back to have my other hip replaced within a year. Since then, four years have passed, and—whatever the X rays show—that other hip is not a source of discomfort. I think the alteration in my eating habits along the lines of the diet indicated above might well have had something to do with that.

"Cures"

Although there are no verified cures for arthritis, I quickly came across plenty of people and companies claiming otherwise. Unfortunately, the lure of the marketplace means that, as with cancer and similar as-yet-incurable diseases, there is no shortage of books, miracle diets, drugs, nutritional compounds, devices, and arcane treatments offering "cures" to arthritis sufferers. Some of these might, indeed, provide a measure of relief for the pain and discomfort of arthritis but are simply overhyped. Some are ineffective but harmless. Some are dangerous. And some are nothing but rip-offs. But none are cures that have been scientifically verified.

It is a measure of the frustration and, in many ways, the desperation that debilitating arthritis can provoke that so many unproven and untested "cures" and treatments enjoy a substantial market, estimated by the FDA at more than $1 billion a year. The scams are legion.

The products and the claims made for them are sometimes dizzying. They range from magnets, copper bracelets, and radon to "therapeutic fasting," snakebites, and bee stings. (These last are offered for sale in "venom" form.) One cure promoted by a number of "health spas"—which, naturally, charge for the service—requires sitting in a uranium mine.

The Food and Drug Administration (FDA) has put out a useful little pamphlet called *Hocus-Pocus as Applied to Arthritis,* published by the *FDA Consumer.* Along with other booklets about arthritis, it is available from the FDA without charge. (Department of Health and Human Services, Food and Drug Administration, Office of Public Affairs, 5600 Fishers Lane, Rockville, MD 20857.)

Traditional folk remedies might likewise provide some relief from pain, but be wary. At the very least, make sure there's nothing harmful in whatever you're putting into your system. I'd also be wary of "proofs" based on anecdotal evidence. That's the easiest kind of evidence to fake. A South African rheumatologist who frequently sends E-mail comments into an arthritis news group on the Internet—he calls himself "Dr. Doc"—tells the following story:

> One or two years ago a celery extract craze hit South Africa with a huge marketing exercise claiming it was tested in Australia and sweeping that continent like a storm with dramatic benefit to all and sundry. Well, I happened to go to Australia in April 1996 to a huge conference on Arthritis and—lo and behold—not a single person was aware of the claims. . . . You patients have something these people want: your wallets.

Some of the most "effective" remedies can be the most dangerous. Many "secret formulas" for relieving arthritis pain, for instance, contain heavy doses of steroids. Short-term, these can often provide seemingly miraculous relief. But taking steroids—especially orally—every day for a period of three to six months could have devastating side effects, not the least of which is undermining the user's autoimmune system to the point where the body would be susceptible to virtually any disease that came along.

The message? To quote a favorite aphorism in the arthritis set: "When someone asks about the theory behind wearing copper bracelets (or some other equally bizarre remedy) to treat arthritis, the answer is simple: The theory is that desperate people will try anything."

The Arthritis Foundation has some good advice along these lines:

Be wary of any product that claims to work for all types of arthritis as well as other health problems. Treatments for the many forms of arthritis vary, and there isn't one treatment known that works on everyone.

Be wary of any product that uses only case histories or testimonials of "satisfied users" as proof that it works. Anecdotes can't replace the assurance of effectiveness and safety that comes from scientific study.

Do not use products that come without printed directions for use or warnings about side effects. All medications approved by the FDA are required to list recommended dosages and precautions on their labels.

Don't use products that don't list contents or that merely describe them as "harmless" or "natural." Some "miracle drugs" are simply more expensive versions of common products like aspirin. Others, labeled as "natural," actually contain powerful drugs that carry the risk of significant side effects. And "natural" doesn't mean it's harmless: Many natural ingredients, such as bee venom, can be dangerous.

Question any treatment that claims to "cure" arthritis. Currently, there is no known cure for most forms of arthritis. If there was such a treatment, many people would know about it, particularly your doctor.

Stay away from products that claim to contain a "secret formula" or are only available from one source. Legitimate scientists share their discoveries so that their results can be reviewed and questioned by other experts in the field. Once proven safe and effective, treatments are made available from many different medical care providers, not just a single person or company.

A word to the wise. Keep in mind the FDA's rule of thumb for evaluating unsubstantiated claims of miraculous cures and permanent relief from arthritis: "If it seems too good to be true, it probably is."

Arthroscopic Surgery

But despite the exercise, the dietary changes, and the medications, my condition continued to worsen. Finally, my family doctor suggested that I see an orthopedic surgeon.

Dr. Stuart Zeman, a Berkeley sports medicine specialist who had been team physician for several professional football teams, took his own X rays, confirmed the arthritis diagnosis, and gave me a cortisone shot to ease the immediate pain. He then recommended arthroscopic surgery for my right knee since it was the joint that was most symptomatic.

Like most people, I am not turned on at the prospect of submitting my body to the whims of the operating table. On the other hand, the alternatives—increasing pain (and immobility) or a steady diet of cortisone shots—didn't register "acceptable" on my quality-of-life meter. The clincher was Zeman's assurance that I'd be back on the tennis courts two months later.

A word about arthroscopic surgery—another one of the technological breakthroughs in modern medicine. Based on the application of miniaturization principles, arthroscopic surgery is probably best known for enabling injured athletes with moderate knee or shoulder damage to return to play within ten days (or even sooner). But it is even more widely used to provide significant relief to arthritis patients. In fact, arthroscopic surgery has become so common—some 1.5 million people have it done every year—that we tend to take it for granted, which is the way it should be.

The procedure is actually called arthroscopy, and it has a dual purpose: to provide the orthopedic surgeon with a direct view inside the ailing joint; and to provide pain relief by removing torn cartilage and other debris and performing minor repairs.

Here's the way it works. After the anesthesia takes effect (in my case it was a general, but it can also be done with an epidural or local anesthesia), the surgeon makes a small incision into which he inserts a pencil-sized instrument called an arthroscope, which has a miniaturized camera on the end. With the arthroscope, the surgeon can project a magnified picture of the joint onto a television monitor. A second incision enables the surgeon to insert miniaturized instruments—scissors, shavers, or drills—into the joint. Then, guiding himself by the image on the television screen, the surgeon uses these instruments to cut away torn tissue or cartilage, smooth down rough spots of cartilage and bone, and perform other, more significant repairs. A third incision enables outflow from the joint of the sterile fluid that is inserted into the joint.

. . .

And that's it: no major incisions, as used to be the case; the blood loss is negligible; a few stitches; relatively rapid recovery; and, in most cases, significant and rapid relief from the preop pain.

Previously, the only way an orthopedic surgeon could clean out or do repairs to an injured joint, let alone examine it directly, was through major invasive surgery on a scale similar to what is now required for a total joint replacement. This meant a hospital stay, a relatively lengthy period of recuperation, and—considering that such surgery was often little more than a stopgap measure—major expense.

Arthroscopic surgery has changed all that. Now the same results can be obtained with an outpatient procedure done in a surgical clinic rather than a hospital, with the patient able to go home the same day. In my case, the operation was performed around 7:30 in the morning and three hours later I was on my way back home. Another plus is that arthroscopic surgery requires a lower level of anesthesia, thereby reducing both the immediate postop recovery time and the risks attendant on any surgery and use of anesthetics. There are the same risks— although they're fewer than with open joint surgery—of infection, blood clots, neurovascular damage, and reactions to anesthesia. (These are estimated at less than 1 percent.)

Although an arthroscopy is fairly minor surgery, there are still a number of important postop steps to take. Reducing the almost inevitable swelling in the knee is one of the first priorities, since this will lessen the pain and enable the recovery process to proceed most rapidly. For that, the main treatment is icing. This should be done several times a day for about twenty to thirty minutes each time. I found the best way to ice my knee was to get into my favorite chair (a recliner is best because it's easy to keep your leg elevated) and watch an old movie on my VCR. And since few of us have an unlimited supply of ice handy, I used a couple of those flexible blue-colored packs that can be refrozen in the freezer compartment of the refrigerator after each use. (They can also be used for heating purposes, either by putting them in boiling water for five minutes or so, or in a microwave oven for one minute.) These packs should always be wrapped in a thin, light towel or some similar cloth and must not be used directly against the skin.

Here are some exercises Dr. Zeman prescribed for me to start doing as soon as I got home.

Quadriceps strengthening: (Quadriceps are the four muscles in the upper leg that join at the kneecap.) Sit on a table with your legs hanging over the edge, a rolled-up towel under your thighs, and a one-pound weight on each ankle. Swing up your left leg until straight and hold for five seconds. Repeat five times. Do the same with the right leg. Do this twice a day for the first week. In the second week, increase the hold time to ten seconds; in the third week, fifteen seconds; and in the fourth week, twenty seconds.

Hamstring strengthening: (Hamstrings are the muscles at the back of the thigh.) You should be lying down in bed on a hard mattress (if you don't already have one, get one) with a small pillow under your head. Bend your knees slightly, then dig your heels forcefully into the bed for a count of six. Relax. Repeat up to ten times. Do this twice a day.

Straight leg lift: Lying flat and keeping the leg straight, raise it eight to twelve inches, hold the position for ten seconds, then relax and bring the leg down. Rest for five seconds. Do this at least ten times. As the knee gets stronger, hold the raised position longer. Aim to get to a total of fifty leg lifts a day. (It is best to do ten or fifteen at a time, especially as the time you hold the position gets longer.)

Heel slide: Bending the knee slightly, slide your heel toward your hip slowly, then straighten. Do this at least ten times, three times a day.

These exercises undoubtedly accelerated my recovery. Two weeks later I was able to take a six-hour coach flight to and from Boston for my daughter's wedding. (I did, however, get the airline to transport me from the curb to the plane in a wheelchair.)

Following my return, I began six weeks of physical therapy (ninety minutes per session three times a week) at a sports medicine center. There I was given electrical stimulation and ultrasound therapy, physical massage, and exercise on a stationary bike and various other pieces of apparatus.

For some people, arthroscopic surgery is of significant benefit. It can put patients back on their feet quickly with varying degrees of relief for varying periods of time. Most important, the procedure buys time. The more one can delay the need for total joint replacement, the better.

For others, like myself, the benefits are temporary. In my case, arthroscopic surgery bought me time and significant—although not total—relief from pain. And Dr. Zeman was true to his word. I was back on the tennis court three months later.

Eighteen months later I had arthroscopic surgery again, this time on my left knee, with similar results. And once again I was back on the tennis court within a couple of months. This time I hooked up with a group of older men, a number of whom had been ranking tennis players in California in their younger years, for regular doubles four times a week. Although not nearly as mobile as I used to be, I fit in well and could compete with the best of them.

This second arthroscopic surgery bought me another eighteen months before my right knee rudely informed me one day that time had run out. Dr. Zeman tried arthroscopic surgery again, but this time it didn't work. Aside from the old arthritis pain, I now had a very focused sharp pain and considerable swelling in the right knee. After draining fluid from the knee, Dr. Zeman took another set of X rays. When these failed to show anything amiss, he suggested another arthroscopy, mainly to see what was going on. But this idea didn't particularly appeal to me.

"In that case," said Dr. Zeman, "I think you're looking at a total knee replacement." But that was a procedure he didn't do.

CHAPTER 2

Total Joint Replacement: Time to Decide

lthough I had been experiencing the discomfort and limitations of advancing arthritis for almost four years, I was not prepared to accept that a total knee replacement was my only solution. I didn't even know then what a total knee replacement was. All I knew was that it sounded pretty drastic. And like most people, I've always looked at surgery of any kind as a final option—something you choose after all alternatives have failed.

Realizing that I had seen only two doctors—my regular GP and Zeman—I began looking around for second opinions and other possibilities. A look through the Yellow Pages yielded the address and phone number of the Arthritis Center, which turned out to be a group of rheumatologists. After taking down my medical history, the doctor I saw made a thorough hands-on physical examination of my legs, hips, and spine, and then took a full set of X rays. His conclusion? I had a fairly advanced case of arthritis that had concentrated in my knees and hips—but also appeared as spurs on my spine.

The rheumatologist recommended medication—more specifically, steroids via a regular series of cortisone injections. But from everything I had heard about steroids, this was not the route I wanted to go.

Cortisone

When they were first developed shortly after World War II, corticosteroids—popularly known as cortisone—were hailed as a new wonder drug. In a landmark test at the Mayo Clinic in 1948, a series of daily injections of the new drug to a group of arthritis patients whose bodies had been deformed and incapacitated by the disease produced a spectacular turnaround in their condition. It was widely thought that a cure for arthritis had at last been found. The doctors who had developed the new miracle drug received the Nobel Prize for Medicine.

The results were so sensational that doctors went on a cortisone binge, prescribing large doses of the drug to their arthritis patients. It was especially effective in treating rheumatoid arthritis, lupus, and several other forms of arthritis. But it wasn't long before the downside of cortisone kicked in. It turned out that the very quality that seemed to make the drug such a prime arthritis fighter was responsible for side effects that, in many instances, were extremely damaging to the body as a whole.

Of course, there are circumstances and conditions in which cortisone might be the only alternative to debilitation or death. Patients with intractable asthma, for instance, might die without it. And many people with rheumatoid arthritis require a great deal of cortisone despite the negative consequences.

Cortisone is so effective because it is a powerful anti-inflammatory agent that can be injected into an arthritic joint. Cortisone can suppress the local inflammation, which is one of the main symptoms of arthritis. Hence the extraordinary short-term results.

But there is a price to be paid for those results if corticosteroids are taken on a regular basis either by injection or orally. They suppress the immune system and, if taken regularly and/or in large doses, undermine the body's defenses. The consequent side effects—really too mild a term for the damage that corticosteroids can do—are numerous.

Perhaps the most serious side effect is that by suppressing the immune system cortisone makes the body much more susceptible to infections and infectious diseases. It can also bring on diabetes, osteoporosis, cataracts, high blood pressure, weight gain, stomach ulcers, easy bruising, muscle weakness, cartilage destruction, acne, and osteonecrosis, in which the bone structure of a joint is dramatically destroyed.

Cortisone can also produce a type of drug dependency. According to Dr. David Pisetsky, author of the *Duke University Medical Center Book of Arthritis* (an excellent and easy-to-read overview of all aspects of arthritis) and a specialist in both immunology and rheumatology:

High doses can cause your own adrenal glands to stop production of cortisol [the body's natural form of cortisone] and can lead to a dependency on the drug. Then, when you come under stress, you may not produce enough cortisol to meet your body's demands. This is called adrenal insufficiency or crisis, a serious, life-threatening condition characterized by weakness, disturbance of salt and water balance, low blood pressure, and eventually shock.

Because of these potential repercussions, many doctors are much more cautious about prescribing cortisone. In general, they seem to agree that something in the neighborhood of four cortisone shots a year is the maximum advisable.

But some physicians continue to prescribe cortisone in ways that could rapidly lead to those serious side effects. One woman with chronic bursitis and osteoarthritis who regularly gets cortisone shots in her hips says that her rheumatologist "is willing to give me the cortisone shots whenever I want. He says it is one of the few ways he can give rapid relief to arthritis patients."

My orthopedic surgeon, Dr. Wolf, includes injections of cortisone among the medications he offers patients who might have an extremely painful joint even though the arthritic changes in the joint might not be very extensive. "When you get to that point," he says, "steroid injections or nonsteroidal anti-inflammatories may provide some relief." But, he adds:

An injection of cortisone in an inflamed knee joint periodically—several times a year—does not have any of the serious negative side effects when compared to long-term daily oral corticosteroid use. I don't have reservations about giving an arthritic patient a cortisone injection in a painful knee or other joint. They often obtain many months of relief. That's what I'd want if it were my knee and I could keep functioning for an extended period of time. I'd want to put off any operation as long as possible as long as I was reasonably comfortable. In fact, you want to delay any joint-replacement surgery as much as possible. Yes, there are some negative effects from cortisone whether taken by injection or orally, but they are dose and frequency related.

But cortisone injections don't work all the time. There seems to be a law of diminishing returns. The first cortisone injection is usually the most effective. The second one may be good. The third may be effective. The fourth one is—well! At some point the disease process has progressed to a point where the knee no longer responds to it. You can't come in every week for an injection. If you start taking it that frequently then you will produce serious negative local and systemic problems. When the injections lose their effect and the pain and deformity are progressing, I usually recommend a total joint arthroplasty.

Alternative Medicine

Although virtually all my doctors are either skeptical or downright cynical about alternative medicine, I next decided to see what homeopathy might have to offer. So I made an appointment at the Heinemann Clinic in Albany, California, to see a homeopathic practitioner who was also an M.D. For an hour and a half, he took down my medical history, my parents' medical histories, my allergies, and so on. He then prescribed a program of vegetable extracts, a homeopathic serum, various enzymes and vitamins, and a diet that was quite similar to—but more detailed than—the one my GP had first given me four years earlier. He also recommended that I stop taking the nonsteroidal anti-inflammatory I had been using. When I asked him if he'd like to look at my X rays, which I had brought along, he said that wasn't necessary. Nor did he physically examine me either for general condition or for joint problems.

I did not understand why my X rays would not be a factor in making a diagnosis or prescribing a program of nutrition and remedies. When I told this story later to people who knew more about homeopathic medicine than I did, they said this was consistent with normal homeopathic procedure, which does not focus on symptoms but on a holistic healing process designed to get at the source of the arthritis.

Well, I'm all in favor of a holistic approach to health. In a culture oriented toward instant gratification, it's not surprising that the tendency—not only by doctors but by most of us—is to deal with health only when we develop the symptoms indicating that something is wrong. After all, despite all the health warnings to the contrary, ours is a culture in which a lot of people practically live on fatty fast-food hamburgers with French fries and far too many people still smoke cigarettes. But although I wish we had a health-care system that placed much greater emphasis on keeping us healthy than on waiting until we get sick, I am thankful for the incredible advances made by medical science in helping us overcome the sicknesses we do get.

So I try to keep an open mind on alternative medicine. I agree with Dr. Wolf—although I'm not sure he meant it the way I took it—when he says that alternative medicine is good for when you're healthy. I also notice that more and more hospitals are getting into what they call "complementary medicine." This might be one of the positive developments coming out of "managed care," since HMOs—in trying to cut costs—seem to be open to the notion that by paying now for alternative approaches they might be able to delay or even avoid expensive treatments (including surgeries) later.

But like many others who have arthritis severe enough to make a joint replacement a serious consideration, I tend to be dubious about the claims of some alternative practitioners when it comes to dealing with major debilitating illnesses such as arthritis in their mature form. And it's not that we're close-minded. But we've heard so many cock-and-bull stories from self-designated "alternative practitioners" offering expensive, long-term courses of treatment as well as a host of expensive remedies that we've become pretty skeptical. Some of these people are clearly crooks and scam artists. Others are undoubtedly well-meaning individuals who believe they're on to something. But sometimes it's hard to tell the difference between them.

Stacy Scott of San Francisco has been through this mill and voices sentiments shared by many of us:

> If my doctor were to call me tomorrow with the news that a cure for RA had been found, my response would be skeptical. I'd expect at the very least to be given a synopsis of the study and its results, and I'd expect to hear some real information on the treatment's dangers, as well as its purported benefits, before I'd consent to try it. I'd expect that if I asked, I'd receive full references for the publication. I would not expect to have my questions answered with nothing except some vague anecdotal reports that someone "felt better" after taking whatever it was. And yet, some proponents of "alternative" medicines all too often seem to expect that we will accept their treatments without demanding evidence, and without the reassurance of information as to the treatments' long-term safety. We are expected to simply try them. There used to be a little Xeroxed poster I'd see pinned to the walls of mailrooms: "I must be a mushroom . . . they keep me in the dark and feed me bulls**t." Well, I feel that way about the claims made

for all too many "alternative" therapies. No, not all doctors answer questions either. But since when did two wrongs make a right?

Perhaps if my arthritis had been diagnosed early enough, a homeopathic approach might have helped ward off or curtail the disease. But by the time I made my way to a homeopath, I already had an advanced form of osteoarthritis. The cartilage in my knees was either all gone or compromised to the point where it was just about useless, and damage to my joints was extensive. I didn't think that this situation was going to be reversed by homeopathic remedies, which, at best, would require long-term treatment. Neither did I have the time, the money, or the inclination to see if the homeopathic treatment would work. So, although I dutifully followed this homeopathic regimen for a while—mostly for want of anything else to do—I didn't have much confidence in it.

This was probably the low point in my years of dealing with arthritis. I remember sitting in my recliner around that time staring out into space. When my wife asked me, "Why are you looking so glum?," all I could say was, "I'm gonna be a cripple the rest of my life."

Cartilage Transplant

At that point I happened on an unexpected ray of hope in the pages of the *New York Times*. (Like many another transplanted New Yorker, I have a tendency not to believe something is real until it is reported in or verified by that arbiter of "all the news that's fit to print.") The ray of hope was an article on experimental work being done with cartilage transplants for people suffering from irretrievable cartilage loss. According to the article, a handful of orthopedic surgeons in the United States had, for the first time, succeeded in transplanting cartilage into the knees of such patients. The article gave the names of five doctors working in this field, one of whom—Dr. Eugene Wolf—was located in San Francisco.

I showed the article to Dr. Frank Anker, a retired physician and my good friend, and asked him how I might go about getting considered for a cartilage transplant.

"Call him up," said Frank.

"Just like that?" I exclaimed.

"Believe me," said Frank. "He'll be happy to talk to you. Doctors developing new procedures are always looking for prospective candidates."

So I followed Frank's advice and, sure enough, was able to reach Dr. Wolf without any difficulty. After thirty minutes on the phone, in which time I went through the story of my arthritis, the various treatments I had undergone, and my present symptoms, Dr. Wolf agreed to see me and we set up an appointment.

Driving over the Bay Bridge on my way from Oakland to San Francisco, I kept returning to Wolf's last words on the phone: "I don't know whether you're a good candidate for a cartilage transplant, but I'm sure I can help you." The words themselves were, of course, encouraging, but there was also something in Dr. Wolf's tone that engendered a sense of confidence that increasingly had been missing from my own usually optimistic disposition.

It didn't take long for Dr. Wolf to dash my hopes of a cartilage transplant. After a manipulative examination of my limbs, one more set of X rays, and close observation of me walking, getting up, turning around, sitting down, and so on, he gave me the news. I didn't have a cartilage transplant in my future. "The typical candidate," Dr. Wolf said, "is someone who has an injury to an otherwise normal knee. . . . You tear the ligament, you tear the meniscal cartilage, but the rest of the knee is normal." Years later, when I was writing this book, he told me, "Your knee was toast."

That was in January 1993. Today cartilage-transplant research has significantly expanded. Dr. Wolf's treatment, like heart and liver transplants, depends on obtaining healthy cartilage from someone who has died (usually younger people killed in an accident). He explains:

The meniscus cartilage is a fibrocartilage, shock-absorbing disk in the knee joint that protects the articular cartilage. Once that articular cartilage is lost, the underlying bone is affected and the disease is irreversible. Current research is also focusing on repairing small, localized, traumatic defects by obtaining cartilage cells from the patient's knee joint.

This is done by using an arthroscope to take a small piece of cartilage from the joint and cultivating it in a laboratory until a few thousand cells grow into millions—a process that usually takes a few weeks. The new cartilage is then injected into the cartilage area in the injured joint. Experiments are also being conducted with other techniques for using the body's own cartilage. Initial results in this area have been promising, but it is too soon to tell whether or not the transplanted cartilage will last long enough to make the surgery viable. Right now it's quite expensive and not covered by most health insurance plans and is of no use once the arthritis process has affected any significant part of the knee joint.

Diagnosis

B
ut before making a diagnosis and recommending a treatment, Dr. Wolf did what he called an "office arthroscopy" on my right knee. Unlike my earlier arthroscopies, this was an arthroscopic examination performed under a local anesthetic in Dr. Wolf's own office. The purpose of the procedure, he said, was to enable him to look at the different compartments of my knee directly— something that could not be done with an X ray or an MRI— and thus make a more accurate diagnosis of my condition than he could otherwise. (The surgery would be so minor, he said, that I would have no difficulty walking or driving home once the anesthesia wore off, roughly thirty minutes after the procedure was done.)

As in arthroscopic surgery, a miniaturized camera attached to an arthroscope is inserted through a small incision in the knee and the image is projected onto a television screen. I was able to watch the screen and see Dr. Wolf conducting his explorations.

Dr. Wolf was trying to determine whether I could get away with a unicompartmental (partial) instead of a total knee replacement. But once he got a good look at my knee, he decided that a partial replacement was not possible.

After that, there was really only one option left: a total knee replacement. The alternatives—a program of steroids, a long-term commitment to "alternative" medicine, which I had become convinced was not going to work, or spending the rest of my life in a wheelchair—were simply unacceptable. Plus, I had found the doctor I was ready to trust with the job.

Finding a Surgeon

Finding a surgeon for your joint replacement is not a simple matter. I came on Wolf almost by accident. Of course, if you're in an HMO or managed-care plan, you will either be assigned to a surgeon or you will choose one from a list the plan provides. (If you find someone you like who is not on the list, you can ask your HMO to cover you, but don't get your hopes up.)

If you're on Medicare, as I am, you've pretty much got your choice, but it might involve some travel or other inconvenience. And in many parts of the country, the choices might be limited. Still, you want to find the surgeon you feel most comfortable with. Your rheumatologist, if you've been seeing one, will most likely recommend someone to you. Or your primary doctor might do so. Your next best bet is to get a recommendation from someone you know who's had a joint replacement and was happy with the surgeon and the outcome.

"If you want a good surgeon," says Craig Norman, director of a program for sports medicine rehabilitation in Oakland, "ask a physical therapist. We see patients from all the surgeons. I see the same good surgeries come from the same good surgeons and I see the same lousy surgeries come from the same lousy surgeons. You see it time and again."

Best is to get the recommendation of another orthopedic surgeon. They know the most about the experience, abilities, and reputations of surgeons in their field. Ask who they would have do their knee or hip replacement if they needed one.

Here are some of the things to look for in a surgeon:

You'll want someone who has a track record with joint-replacement surgery and with your particular joint. I went with Dr. Wolf for my knee replacements even though his particular specialty is shoulders because he had considerable experience with knees and because I developed confidence in him. Later on, when I needed a total hip replacement, I stayed with Dr. Wolf because he told me he had done many hip replacements and because I had gotten such good results with my knees.

Look for someone who will level with you and give you informative answers to your questions. All too many doctors act as though patients are simpletons who need to be spoon-fed as little information as possible. This isn't just a matter of style. A fully knowledgeable and independent-minded patient will do better than one who unquestioningly accepts whatever the surgeon says. That patient will also be more likely and in a better position to take responsibility for his or her own recovery.

Find out something about your surgeon's training, medical school attended, and internship. Don't be embarrassed about asking your surgeon these kinds of questions. And once the recommendation for joint-replacement surgery has been made, don't hesitate to get a second opinion.

Check out the hospital where the surgery will be performed. Is orthopedic surgery one of its specialties? Does it offer joint-replacement patients preop classes? (A growing number of hospitals are doing that these days. See chapter 4 for more on this subject.)

Finally, make sure your surgeon and the hospital will accept Medicare's designated price. (Most surgeons will, but don't take it for granted.) Medicare assigns a price for each service and will pay 80 percent of that price. You're responsible for the other 20 percent unless you have what's popularly known as Medigap insurance. Also, you're responsible for the cost of your first day in the hospital unless, again, you have Medigap. For me, Medigap coverage was a godsend. The total cost of my three joint replacements was roughly $100,000, of which Medicare paid $80,000. (The total would be higher today.) So I would have had to come up with $20,000 without the secondary coverage. Since my Medigap policy was costing about $900 a year at that point, I came out well ahead. This is to say nothing of other procedures my secondary insurance has covered.

Knees and Hips: A Brief User's Guide

To understand what's involved in a total joint replacement, we'll need a quick course in the nature of the two joints where replacement surgery is both the most common and the most advanced: the knee and the hip.

The medical shorthand that talks about a joint replacement is somewhat misleading because it suggests that a joint is a single object. In fact, a joint is a structure made up of several parts. A knee, for instance, consists of three bones: the lower portion of the thigh bone (called the femur), which runs from the hip to the knee; the upper portion of the shin bone (called the tibia), which runs from the ankle to the knee; and the kneecap (called the patella).

Then there's cartilage—the firm, rubbery material that covers the places where the bone comes into contact with other bones. (These are called articular surfaces; the cartilage that covers these surfaces is called articular cartilage to differentiate it from other types of cartilage, such as meniscal cartilage, which is also found in the knee.)

In addition, there is a complex of ligaments, muscles, and tendons that function as flexible cables, giving the knee support, strength, and mobility. These are enclosed in a capsule lined by a thin material called the synovial membrane, which releases a special fluid that lubricates the knee.

All this constitutes the knee, the largest, most complicated, and most used joint in your body.

The most conspicuous property of the knee is its flexibility. This is what enables us to walk, run, bend, twist, squat, and perform a broad range of other physical functions. At the same time, the knee is a major weight-bearing joint. Watch the knees when weight lifters make the transition from their first lift (waist high) to the second (at the chest) to the third (over the head), and you will get some idea of how the combination of flexibility and weight bearing makes the knee such a significant joint in the body's functioning. None of this would be possible without cartilage.

Compared to the knee, a hip is a relatively simple joint. Also a main weight-bearing joint, a hip has two main parts: a ball and a socket. The ball, which is situated at the head of your thighbone (the femur) fits into a rounded socket in the pelvic bone. Like the knee, the bone surfaces of the ball and socket are covered with the extremely smooth articular cartilage that covers the bone surfaces at the knees, thus allowing for easy, fluid motion.

Partial Knee and Hip Replacements

Even if your ability to move has been severely limited and your knee or hip has been extremely painful, you still might not need a total joint replacement. Your orthopedic surgeon might find that only one area in the joint has been affected and the rest of the joint might be good for another ten years or so. Under those circumstances a partial (unicompartmental) joint replacement might be called for.

But even with X rays, MRIs, and diagnostic arthroscopy, the surgeon might not know for sure whether you need a partial or total joint replacement until your joint is opened up on the operating table.

This was the case when I observed a knee-replacement operation myself. The patient was a seventy-three-year-old woman who already had undergone a right total knee arthroplasty performed by Dr. Wolf. Going into the operating room, Dr. Wolf told me he wasn't sure whether he would be doing a partial or total replacement on her left knee and that the decision would be made on the operating table. It was only after her knee had been fully opened and the condition of the entire knee evaluated that Dr. Wolf decided on a total knee replacement. But it was a close call. Dr. Wolf finally opted for a total rather than a partial because, he told me, the patient would probably need a total anyway within a few years and there was no good reason to subject her to an additional surgery.

In the course of talking to other joint-replacement patients, I came across two cases of partial hip replacements.

When thirty-eight-year-old Bill Kennedy of San Jose learned that he had a benign tumor in the head of his femur, he wound up with a partial hip replacement. Nine months later he wrote, "My doctor thinks I'm doing great, but since I was active up until my surgery, the result is not as satisfactory as it would be for someone crippled from the pain of arthritis."

In the case of eighty-one-year-old Edward Shineman of New York City, the problem was a fracture of the femur as the result of an accident on the tennis court. Three months after getting a partial hip replacement, Shineman wrote: "I'm able to walk one or two miles, but there's no indication when I can resume tennis." I like that attitude, especially the "when" rather than an "if." I bet he will, too.

Another surgical alternative to a joint replacement is called an osteotomy. This operation is usually done to correct a pain-producing deformity; for example, if the patient is extremely bowlegged and all the stresses and strains are on the inside part of the knee. Dr. Wolf describes this procedure:

A wedge of bone is removed—usually from the tibia, although it can also be out of the femur—just like if you were taking a wedge out of a tree to make it fall in a particular direction. Then we close the wedge and since the weight is then shifted to that part of the knee that has some cartilage on it, your knee is now straight. But you have to have a specific deformity and some good cartilage to shift onto. You didn't have that.

Similarly with a hip. Where deformity is producing the problems, correcting the deformity can sometimes correct the problem. The problem with most hips and most knees, however, is that the problem isn't in just one area. It's global. The whole thing just wears out.

When Is It Time for a Joint Replacement?

When Dr. Wolf recommended that I have a total knee replacement, I thought back to the rheumatologist I had seen earlier who had advised against the operation because, among other things, I was too young. Well, when you're sixty-seven—as I was then—and someone says you're too young for anything, you can't help but admire their perspicacity. But then when it dawns on you that you're being told to live with increasing pain, decreasing mobility, and a life of frustration and loss of independence, you might have second thoughts about that dubious compliment.

I did, and I concluded that age should be, at most, a secondary factor in deciding on a joint replacement. Number one should be quality of life. True, knee or hip replacement is major surgery. But when pain and immobility have diminished your quality of life to the point where it has become unacceptable, you are ready for a joint replacement. Those doctors who say you're too young usually say so because the traditional view is that joint replacements last only ten to fifteen years and a second replacement is more difficult. But if you are still willing to submit to major surgery after being told about the risks and limitations, then I think your surgeon should accommodate you.

Besides, this is a new and rapidly developing field. Both surgical techniques and prostheses have improved since those first averages were compiled. No one knows for sure how long the new prostheses will last, but it seems that they're being made better and stronger. And who knows what changes there will be ten or fifteen years down the road? So why surrender the best years of your life to constant pain and increasing immobility?

In time, I was to hear this same story from many other arthritis sufferers. Forty-one-year-old Jeff Solka, who has been battling osteoarthritis for four years, wrote me after being told he wasn't ready for a hip replacement: "Best I have heard, you have to crawl into the Rheumies' office for a couple of years in excruciating pain before they will even consider you for a joint replacement."

Generally, the reason for this "too young" response is that many doctors are reluctant to recommend a procedure in which the patient is likely to outlive the prosthesis. Certainly, a doctor should make sure that the patient is fully informed about any procedure: the benefits, the risks, the alternatives, and, in this case, the life expectancy of the prosthesis. But once it's been established that there are no acceptable alternatives except a life of increasing pain and physical limitations, the decision should be up to the patient, not the doctor.

This is especially true for people with rheumatoid arthritis, since they tend to be much younger. Asking someone in his twenties or thirties who is living with a crippling disease to wait until he is in his sixties before getting a desired joint replacement is the same as condemning him to a lifetime of suffering.

Rose Marie Balan of British Columbia has rheumatoid arthritis so severe that when she was twenty-five her surgeon agreed to perform a total knee replacement. Three years later she had a hip replaced, and the following year her other knee. Several years later, her first knee was replaced again. In 1998, when she was forty-three, Rose wrote: "Since then, I have had no further replacements. So if the concern is that a joint will not last, mine have lasted for more than thirteen years. A benefit of being younger when you have the surgery is that you recuperate faster. In my opinion, there is no real benefit to waiting when you are in constant pain. If there is no longer a quality of life, then it is time regardless of your age."

I think if some of these timorous doctors found them- selves in our situation they'd change their tune pretty quickly—especially if they faced the prospect of being unable to pursue their careers.

When, later on, I asked Dr. Wolf why he had recommended that I have a joint replacement after others had suggested I wait, he said:

I knew what your goals were. That's the most important thing. What does the patient want? I could see you were going to be unhappy with the low level of activity you'd have without a knee replacement. I don't recommend waiting when the patient's quality of life has markedly deteriorated and has reached the point where he or she finds it unacceptable. Then a lot of patients—like you—are very anti-steroid. So I can't say you must have a steroid

injection. I know it won't cure your knee. I know it'll only
give you temporary relief from the pain. I know you'll be
back in weeks or months and tell me it's hurting again. So
I replace your knees and you're happy. That's what it's all
about. I want to make people happy. I want people coming
back saying, "This is great! I wanna write a book about
this!" I want people coming back and saying, "Thank you!
The pain is gone." I don't want them coming back saying,
"Oh, it's hurting again" or "The medications are tearing up
my stomach" or "I need another injection."

Well, Dr. Wolf definitely read me right. And I'm glad he did.
But that doesn't mean you should rush into a joint replacement
at the first signs of arthritic pain and stiffness. A joint replacement requires major surgery with all the risks surgery entails.
It should be seriously considered only when the pain and lack
of mobility significantly interfere with your ability to function
and your quality of life. Not so long ago, people like myself
didn't even have a choice. Now we do. Joint-replacement
surgery has provided an alternative—at least for some of us—
to an increasingly painful and constricted life.

One of the best facilities for joint replacements in the
United States is the Department of Orthopaedic Surgery at
the University of Iowa Hospitals and Clinics. Dr. John
Callaghan, head of the department, gives the following
advice to family doctors regarding painful hips, although the
principle clearly applies to knees as well:

The primary care physician should refer the patient to an
orthopedist when the physician and/or the patient is concerned that the increase in pain and decrease in mobility are
functionally disabling and markedly limiting the patient's
lifestyle, even with nonsurgical therapy. When patients
experience regular, daily, moderate severe hip pain that

limits their ability to walk comfortably for more than several blocks, interferes with daily activity (ability to climb stairs, bathe and dress, get in and out of cars and chairs), and is not relieved by analgesics and NSAIDs, the patient should consider the risks and benefits of surgery. (*Journal of the American Medical Association*, August 14, 1996)

There might be other considerations in delaying a joint replacement. A surgeon will understandably be reluctant to operate on someone who is extremely overweight and might insist that you get some of that excess weight off. And there might be other physical conditions that make surgery dangerous.

Unfortunately, however, some patients who need a joint replacement, are ready for it, want it, and have no health conditions preventing it, still have difficulty getting one. One reason, of course, is cost. For someone without health insurance, the total cost of a typical knee or hip replacement (that includes the surgeon's fee, hospital charges, anesthesia, doctor visits, physical therapy, and so forth) will be somewhere between $35,000 and $45,000. And that's beyond the reach of many individuals.

Mairabet, a full-time church employee in Boston, "began to have some of the 'minor' aches and pains of arthritis" in the 1980s. As her condition worsened, she had cortisone shots, tried "enormous doses" of NSAIDs, and consulted with more doctors than she cares to remember. By 1996 she was at the point where she was willing to consider a joint replacement. But her job does not provide her with health insurance coverage. In response to an E-mail note I sent advising her to consult an orthopedic surgeon, she wrote:

As for an operation, I think the timing is out of the question because I am now a single person and self-supporting which means there would be nobody to pay the bills if I were laid up for any length of time, and then for a few weeks afterward probably could not drive my car to work. My hope is to treat the osteoarthritis for the time being with whatever is most advisable and helpful, and then to get the operation(s) done when I go on Medicare. In 1997, I will be 60 and thus not so very many years away from Medicare.

Some patients in HMOs tell of long delays—first in getting approval for a joint replacement and then in having it scheduled. This is not surprising. With HMOs giving doctors incentives for not recommending expensive treatments and disincentives if they do, it is virtually inevitable that thousands of people who need and want joint replacements are going to face extensive delays, if not outright denial of authorization. I guess that's the price we pay for buying into the notion that decent health care is not a right that society should ensure for everyone.

But it pays to put up a fight.

Take the case of Chris Barnsley, who wrote to me in April 1996:

I am 37 years old and have Ankylosing Spondylitis. I have been having severe problems with my left hip for the last few years. It has affected all aspects of my life and my quality of life is steadily going down the tubes. I take at least six and as much as nine Tylenol three times a day to manage the pain. . . . I go to physiotherapy three times a week for my hip and neck. (I have less than 30 degrees mobility in my neck, but it is finally pain free.) Even after Cortisone shots I have bad days where I can hardly walk and I limp even on good days. I also use a cane quite often.

The last time I saw my doctor (about a year ago) I told him

I wanted a hip replacement. But he said I was too young and that the new hip would only last 15 years at the most. He suggested continuing with the Cortisone. I am afraid for my job, my relationship with my wife, my ability to be able to have a life in general. My employer and my wife have been great about this, but I am getting to be a real burden to both of them and I want it to stop. I want my life back.

I wrote to Chris and told him how my three joint replacements had helped me. I suggested that he speak to his doctor again and emphasize the issues relating to the loss of quality of life.

That was the last I heard from Chris for six months. Then, on October 30, the following note showed up in my E-mail:

You might be interested to know that I had my total hip replacement on October 18 and I am now home and recovering. I took your advice and discussed quality of life with my doctor and the next thing I knew I was scheduled for the operation. All is going well. I was in less pain immediately after the surgery than I was just before I went in. I have been looking forward to my new life and have been telling others what you told me. "Quality of life is the most important thing in the world."

Karen Sandy, my physical therapist, contends that once you know you're going to need a joint replacement, you're better off doing it sooner rather than later. After working with and observing thousands of hip- and knee-replacement patients, she believes:

Hip-replacement patients who have waited a very long time before going ahead with the surgery—maybe they are ill or afraid, maybe they had other things that had to be done first, maybe they had no one in the family who could help them at the time—have a more difficult recovery because generally the whole body is in a weaker state. They haven't been able to be as active and the muscles around the hip have to be weaker. The same would hold true with knee replacements. People who have waited a long time generally have a harder time trying to get the knee strong, to move it. Remember you're trying to get flexion, range of motion, trying to get extension, your muscles have to be strong enough to pull against the tightness that you have. And if you're going into the surgery with a very weak musculature around the knee, it's just going to take that much longer to recover.

Physical therapist Craig Norton says, "Doing this for almost twenty-five years, I have found that the younger people are when they have their knee replacements, the more successful they seem to be."

Different Strokes for Different Folks

Of course, not everyone who might benefit from a joint replacement is psychologically ready for surgery. Most people wait until the pain becomes unbearable and their quality of life has deteriorated to the point where they have been forced to surrender all but the most sedentary activity. And even then, some will not consider a joint replacement. When I asked Dr. Wolf about this, he said:

After being in this profession twenty-five years I can pretty quickly assess who is going to go the conservative pathway regardless of the situation. And then there are patients who are suffering so much not only physically but emotionally with the changes impacting their lives that they're willing to take the risks of surgery—and there are risks—in order hopefully to maintain a lifestyle that makes them happy. Because when you get down to it, being happy is really what it's about. Some people are happy sitting in a chair. Some people take vacations to sit on a chair on the beach. And some people take vacations to run a marathon every day. Or wind-surf or some kind of nonstop activity. They're happy with that. That person is a different patient. You're that kind of patient. You wanted to play tennis again and everything that represents. And when you're dealing with patients, it's not the X ray that settles the issue. It's what the patient wants. You want to go through with a big operation with the risks of that operation to continue a lifestyle, well, that's what you have to do. Somebody else, he plays checkers, he sits on a bench, plays with his tiles, and he's satisfied.

Karen Sandy, my physical therapist, believes that people who have joint replacements are generally a healthy population because they have opted for an elective surgery. "They are people," she says, "who usually have been physically active—at least up until the time that the arthritis got so bad that their activities were curtailed." In this sense, she considered me "a typical joint-replacement patient."

And in the vast majority of cases, a joint replacement will enable those who could most benefit from it to overcome the anxiety, fear, and natural reluctance all of us have when faced with the prospect of invasive surgery.

Still, fear of surgery holds many people back. No one, of course, is thrilled at the prospect of a major operation. And so long as we think there's a chance of avoiding it, most of us will. But if I had a dollar for every joint-replacement patient who has said, "I only wish I had the surgery earlier," I'd be planning a vacation in Hawaii.

Carol Downing of Port Orange, Florida, saw how her father paid the price for stalling after a hip replacement was recommended to him:

> My dad had osteoarthritis in his hip from an injury and put off surgery for years. How he suffered. . . . By the time he decided to finally get the surgery done, the hip was too far gone. The surgery he ended up having was far more serious than the one he originally anticipated. On top of that, he had developed osteoarthritis in his other hip because of the strain on it for so many years. That one he did have replaced.
>
> I have rheumatoid arthritis and I'm sure the time will come when surgery will be an issue. Maybe it's because I've witnessed the effects of procrastination, but I will take the advice of my good doctors and move ahead.

One January day in 1997 I came across an interesting interchange in my favorite arthritis news group on the Internet. A forty-four-year-old man who had been suffering from rheumatoid arthritis for five years acknowledged that a knee replacement would probably help him but expressed a fear of surgery, writing:

> I take prednisone, mtx, plaquinel, azulfidine, amytryptaline and oruvail. I have had about 10 cortisone injections into my knee, but the last one didn't help at all. The pain is constant, keeping me awake at night, so it hurts even when I'm not walking. Is surgery my only option?

Immediately following was a reply from Joan Stuart, which I recommend to anyone wrestling with the "Should I?" or "Shouldn't I?" question.

Don't be frightened of knee surgery. I have had a total knee replacement and a total hip replacement in the same leg and have never regretted it. I have severe rheumatoid arthritis and am on many of the same drugs you are. I was only in hospital for four days after my knee replacement (18 months ago). I had quite a bit of pain initially after the operation but the pain I had before was much worse. My post-op pain gradually diminished and I was off crutches after 6 weeks. I now walk without any aids and am pain free. It is wonderful. I put off the operation for years and wish I had done it in the beginning. I could have saved myself years of unnecessary pain. Go for it and good luck!!!

CHAPTER 3

Not by Statistics Alone: Patient Experiences

U ntil recently, surgery was not seriously considered as a way to treat arthritis. Even today, most books on arthritis written for the general public—and there are dozens—have little to say about the possibility of joint replacements. One popular book—its cover claims "more than 400,000 copies sold"—devotes more than fifty pages to a detailed discussion of medications (five pages on steroids alone) for treating what it acknowledges is an "incurable" disease and less than a single page to joint replacements. Another also offers fifty pages of advice on arthritis medications and thirty more on "Other Forms of Treatment" but little more than a page on joint replacements.

Still, much of this literature is useful—as far as it goes. These books generally provide helpful information on the nature of arthritis, how to adjust one's life to the condition, and the role of exercise, cortisone, nonsteroidal anti-inflammatory drugs, and nutrition in managing the pain and making life as bearable as possible. But they provide minimal information about joint replacements, which is what I was looking for.

One clue to the short shrift given joint replacements by many writers can be found in the remark made by an aggressively assertive rheumatologist on the Internet. "Orthopods [meaning orthopedic surgeons] are not diagnosticians," he wrote, "they are hackers who cut and chisel."

Is there a whiff of sour grapeshot in that salvo? Rheumatologists used to rule the roost in the field of arthritic medicine, but what even many of their partisans now admit is that "most people who have this surgery are thrilled with the results." As a result, the "hackers and chiselers" have won new and widespread respect for developing the most promising new treatments for arthritis sufferers and, indeed, for revolutionizing the field.

Not that prospective replacement surgery is risk-free. Dr. Wolf was frank about the risks when he first suggested I might be happy with a joint replacement. But he also took me through the whole procedure, showed me the kind of prosthesis I'd have put into my knee, and later my hip, and gave me a pretty good idea of what to expect after surgery. And I could have put off the operation. I had lost a lot of mobility and was frustrated at my inability to pursue those activities I had always enjoyed, but—except for the two-month period leading up to my hip replacement in March 1994, which, as my grandmother used to say, "I wouldn't wish on my worst enemy"—the pain was not unbearable. (To paraphrase the old joke, it only hurt when I walked.)

When I talked over the decision with my wife, however, I told her that Dr. Wolf made me feel I had found a way out of the morass I was in and that I was inclined to go ahead with the surgery immediately. That's a decision I've never had either regrets or second thoughts about.

And so I became another of the several million patients undergoing total hip and knee replacements in the United States alone since the first total joint replacements were done in the late 1960s. Of these, more than 90 percent were "successful."

How Do You Measure Success?

That word *successful* needs some explaining, however. Out of 100 total knees or hips one year after surgery, Dr. Wolf says the success rate would be in the 96 to 98 percent range; that is, for those patients, the new joint would be working, they would have at least 80 percent reduction of pain, and they would be functioning normally. At six years it might be 92 percent and at ten years it might be 90 percent. Even if your joint subsequently needed a major overhaul (and possibly another replacement), most people would probably consider that their surgery was a success if they had obtained ten additional years of functionality on what used to be a severely painful and fundamentally nonfunctional hip or knee.

A lot has to do with your expectations going in. One of the keys to success is preparing the patient. Dr. Wolf says:

I'm going to make you better, but I'm not going to give you a normal knee. Although I'll take away a lot of the pain, it's rare that a patient will be absolutely, totally pain-free. But if you can be relieved of 80 percent of your pain and function now with 20 percent of your pain, chances are you'll be pretty happy. You'll have some limitation of motion and you won't have the same kind of flexibility as a normal knee; nor the same kind of what we call "proprioception"—which means the sense of it being a normal knee. But when you compare your preoperative with your postoperative status you'll have to say, "I'm a lot better and it was worth doing it."

Success is not simply a statistic. It's countless stories of individuals resuming careers and regaining self-esteem, of confidence replacing despair, children regaining parents, and elders regaining the dream of (relatively) painless golden years lived with dignity. Above all, it is rescue from lives that would otherwise be blighted by pain, deformity, lack of mobility, and loss of independence.

In my case—since I had three joint replacements within months of each other—I really couldn't measure success until after the third. Even so, I enjoyed a significant improvement in my quality of life even after the first operation (my right knee). Two months after surgery I could walk without a cane, and I'd regained much of my earlier self-sufficiency. And, despite some stiffness, the pain was 90 percent gone. But that was just one down and two to go. I was still a long way from the goal I had marked on my private barometer—playing tennis once again. I knew that goal would probably not be on my agenda until all my ailing joints had been replaced.

Even as my new knee kicked in, the other knee developed what I can only conclude was a severe case of jealousy and let me know in no uncertain terms that it wanted attention. Then my left hip got on the bandwagon. It was only after these were also replaced that my recovery really shifted into high gear. There's more to a successful joint replacement, however, than the operation. Your orthopedic surgeon has a crucial role to play, of course. But so do you. Later on I will talk about the role of mental attitude and physical therapy in this process. For now, it's enough to note—as I pointed out in the introduction to this book—that although I can't do everything I used to do ten years ago (who can?), I have my life back again and I *am* playing tennis.

The significant thing about my "success" is that it is not unusual, let alone unique.

How do you measure success? The bottom line is whether there is a qualitative improvement for each joint-replacement patient in four critical areas: relief from pain; renewed mobility; independence; and a drastic change for the better in the individual's quality of life.

Joint replacements do not cure arthritis. But they can neutralize and overcome the most crippling effects of that disease. Here's what joint replacements have meant in the lives of some people who went through the process after trying all the alternatives, agonizing over the decision, overcoming their own fears and anxieties, and eventually biting the bullet.

What's striking about most of these stories is the determination shown by so many patients to regain their independence and the elation they feel in telling others of their experience.

The Odyssey of Elayne Jones: "I only wish I had the surgery earlier"

Elayne Jones is the tympanist with the San Francisco Opera orchestra. She was sixty-seven when, after complaining of hip pain, she was diagnosed as having osteoarthritis. That was in 1995. Despite increasing pain and decreasing mobility, she stalled on having her hip replaced because the pain was still bearable and she didn't want to take time off from her job.

Elayne was the first black musician—male or female—to hold a position as principal player in any major symphony orchestra in the world when she joined the San Francisco Symphony. Elayne is a fighter. She never would have gotten or kept her job if she weren't. And she was sure she could find a way to beat the arthritis just as she has beaten most of the obstacles she has encountered in her life. Most people who have been told they need a joint replacement can probably identify readily with her efforts to avoid surgery, although I don't know how many would have tried all the things she did.

When I first learned I had arthritis, I couldn't believe it. Then, as people began to mention the possibility of getting a hip replacement, I decided there had to be a better way. First I went to a chiropractor for a couple of months. I was given special vitamins which, I was told, would "heal" and strengthen the bones. No improvement. Then I was recommended to a "deep tissue therapist" who also used chiropractic methods. He also believed that the mind and body worked together, so at each session we spent a half-hour talking and then one hour on the table. I felt good but the pain really didn't get any better. In the meantime I had read about Glucosamine Sulfate and started taking it. I also took Evening Primrose Oil tablets.

I was then recommended to a highly acclaimed preventive care doctor whose office happened to be near my house. I went to him and he listened to me, but he never touched me. However he said I was eating "too much fruit." I had to stop eating fruit. He gave me alkaline to drink twice a day. He also thought that the problem might be due to a lack of hormones. He suggested I take progesterone. I balked at that and fortunately I had the good sense not to take it. I finally stopped going to him because everything he advised me to take I had to buy from him. One item was far more expensive than at Real Foods. I just felt he was in it for the money and his place was like a factory with a steady stream of people going in and coming out.

I began swimming three times a week thinking that the exercise would ease the pain. I returned to the Deep Tissue therapist only to find that I was having more pain from my sessions with him. Although the pain was steadily getting worse, I kept believing that someone would find the answer to relieve the pain.

The last person I went to said he believed that the bone could heal itself with the proper nutrients. So he sold me Chinese herbs and took me off all kinds of foods which he said were the cause of the pain. I don't know which was worse, the deprivation of the foods I loved or the pain. Whichever, I was miserable. I also developed a terrible rash all over my body. I didn't know the cause but I suspected the Chinese herbs. One day, after having gone to him for a month-and-a-half, he gave me an acupuncture treatment which totally crippled me. I never went back. Each person I went to had another theory about how I could get better, putting me and my living patterns through their beliefs.

I felt my whole body was in a state of collapse. Nothing made me feel good while the pain continued to get worse. I first had to give up tennis. (I used to play pretty vigorous singles and doubles three or four times a week and had won a number of tournaments.) Although I love to dance and entertain, I couldn't do either. I stopped inviting people to my home because cooking and shopping became too difficult. I stopped going to the theater and attending concerts because sitting for long stretches became too uncomfortable.

The worst part was that I didn't expect the pain to get so severe. Finally, I had to stop working. I just couldn't get to work. I had never missed a day with the orchestra in almost 25 years, so that was really traumatic. I could hardly walk and, by then, I was taking 2400 mg of Motrin a day. At that point I had to acknowledge that if I ever wanted to get back to work or have something resembling a normal life I'd have to go the surgery route.

On November 27, 1996, Elayne had her right hip replaced by Dr. Curtis Kiest at Kaiser Hospital in San Francisco. Two weeks later she sent me an E-mail note:

I feel marvelous. My physical therapist is very impressed with my strength and progress. I only wish I had the surgery earlier. Everyone took advantage of my denial as to what was wrong and tried to capitalize on it. It cost me thousands of dollars and undue pain. Well-meaning people should understand that once you've got osteoarthritis, the holistic route, however much we might like to go that way, isn't going to help. Unfortunately, the only cure seems to be surgery. I think I went through enough to prove that.

Doris Stokes:
"No pain since six hours after the surgery"

Fifty-three-year-old Doris Stokes of Fort Smith, Arkansas, calls herself "a walking commercial for total knee replacements." I can understand why. As a result of osteoarthritis, Doris's left knee had "been in pain for nine years and in extreme pain for seven months." In June 1996, at the Sparks Medical Center in Fort Smith, her knee was replaced by Dr. James Long. Before surgery, she says,

I could not do many of the activities I was used to doing. I couldn't walk but a short distance without sitting down for a few minutes. I couldn't even walk in the grocery store long enough to do my shopping. Standing was worse than walking.
I was ready for relief. I asked for the surgery and was thrilled to have it. I was on an emotional high because I had

the chance to be pain free. Well, I have had no pain since six hours after the surgery.

I had my first physical therapy the next morning around 10 a.m. They taught me how to get in and out of bed and walked me from the bed to the door of my room. That afternoon they started me on quad sets. The next day they walked me down the hall approximately 25 feet and brought me back in a wheelchair and started me on a new exercise: a straight leg lift. Over the next couple of days I increased the holding time on both the quad sets and the leg-lift and increased my hall walk to 200 feet.

After a week at home, I was able to completely take care of myself. I bathed myself, dressed myself, went to the table to eat. I even cooked some meals after a couple of weeks. The one thing I couldn't do was carry things since I was using a walker. *

I used a walker for six weeks and then a cane for two weeks. I kept misplacing my cane, so the doctor said that was a sign that I didn't need it. Shortly afterwards I went to Las Vegas, walked all over the Strip and have not stopped walking since. And I still do the stretching, lifting and bending exercises once a day.

This was four months after her left knee was replaced. At the same time, Doris told me that she was scheduled to have her right knee replaced in three months. "As a result of the arthritis," she wrote, "both my legs were very bowed. My left leg is now straight and my right one will be soon."

And, in her last note to me, she says it is.

---

* I solved this problem by attaching a plastic basket to the front of my walker. That way I could transport light objects—a book, a sandwich, the morning paper—from one place to another. You've just got to be careful not to put too much weight in the basket or it will tip the walker over. My physical therapist, Karen Sandy, recommends using a tea cart to carry various objects. You can push the cart ahead of you while using the walker.

John Kiefer:
"Don't let the doctor tell you you're too young"

J ohn Kiefer of Norfolk, Virginia, is a former career Marine Corps officer who was found "unfit for further duty" because of a degenerating hip brought on by osteoarthritis. First diagnosed in 1990, when he was thirty-seven, John's condition quickly deteriorated.

I had to stop running, hiking, karate (I've practiced it since I was twelve) and snow-skiing. I was unable to go for even short walks, especially my favorite pastime of walking my 136-pound German Shepherd.

Fortunately, John stayed in the service long enough to qualify for regular retirement status. Thus, when his left hip was replaced in January 1996, the surgery was done at the Portsmouth Naval Hospital in Portsmouth, Virginia. The operation was performed by Drs. Russell, Cellos, and Lewis, all U.S. Navy officers.

The surgery went well. Although John faithfully followed the special instructions regarding hip replacements, he admits, "I was not very committed to the physical therapy." Happily his wife was, so he did his leg lifts, butt crunches, flutter kicks, and the rest of his prescribed exercises. At his doctor's suggestion, he used a walker for the first six weeks.

The Doc said that he prefers a walker over crutches not just for the added stability but because it signals people around you to get out of the way better than crutches do.

In November 1996, John wrote to tell me he was doing fine.

No more karate, skiing, jogging. But after my hip started going bad, I couldn't do those things anyway. Now I can enjoy long walks again without even a limp.

His thoughts for anyone facing the prospect of a joint replacement?

A supportive spouse really helps. If you're adept at using the Internet, do some research. Ask your doctor questions. Don't let him tell you you're too young. Listen to him, of course, but you must make this decision based on your quality of life.

Dietmar Hartl:
"The hip replacements were like being reborn"

Although most joint-replacement patients suffer from osteoarthritis, people with other forms of arthritis can be candidates for joint-replacement surgery. One of the most crippling of the arthritic diseases is ankylosing spondylitis (AS), a chronic inflammatory disease that particularly attacks the sacroiliac joints, the joints that connect the spine to the pelvic bones. Since your hip socket is at the other end of the pelvic bone, the hips are often affected. In advanced cases of AS, a process of ossification often occurs in which the spine is fused and becomes stiff and inflexible.

Dietmar Hartl of British Columbia has had AS since the age of eleven. (The disease is most prevalent among young men, although it can last a lifetime.) He writes:

As a result of the spondylitis, both my hips were totally fused and immobile so that they felt as hard as rock and I was stuck inside! My quality of life went to just about zero. I was house-bound, pain-bound, depressed, unable to work or swim or even walk. At times I got so scared that I thought I could no longer breathe.

In 1985, when he was thirty, Hartl had both hips replaced. "It was like being reborn," he says. "It was so powerful being able to walk again, I cried."

Elizabeth "Betita" Martinez: "We gave each other a high five after the second surgery"

Betita Martinez is a well-known Chicana writer, teacher, and political activist. In 1974, her book *Viva la Raza* won the Jane Addams Children's Book Award. Among her other books is *500 Years of Chicano History*, a bilingual pictorial history widely used by schools, youth groups, and community organizations. In 1968, she began the Chicano activist newspaper *El Grito del Norte* and edited it for its first five years. She has also written for *The Nation*, where she was books and arts editor, and the *Village Voice*, and was, for a time, an editor at Simon & Schuster.

Betita, who also lives in the Bay Area, has been a good friend for many years; and when she had her first hip replacement in 1993, at the age of sixty-seven, I was having my first knee replacement. So we monitored each other's woes and triumphs intensely. In 1997, Betita had her other hip replaced. Both were done at Kaiser Permanente in San Francisco by Dr. Gordon Engel, chief of orthopedics.

Although her recovery was slower and somewhat more painful than mine, she has regained her mobility, is living relatively pain-free, and, as always, remains as busy and active as any thirty-year-old. Looking back on the experience, she says:

A joint replacement is usually a striking example of the wonders of the human body, for which we can all be grateful. Along with that gratitude comes being thankful that I live in a time when joint replacements are possible. If I had lived earlier, I would have been in a wheelchair for the past four years and the rest of my life. Joint replacement seems to me one of Western medicine's finest achievements. If you can control pain without surgery, of course that's preferable—but sometimes it's no longer possible. I also had the advantage of a surgeon I had known for almost twenty years whose opinion I valued. When we gave each other a high five after the second surgery, I felt we were celebrating his skill, my survival, and the wonders of the human body—all at once.

Still waiting to be accomplished is a society where everyone, thanks to having good health insurance, can be freed from pain and immobility as happened to me. Now that will call for the all-time big high five!

Them Bones
Will Rise Again

The decision to go ahead with a joint replacement was a major turning point in my life. It set me on a journey that would enable me to regain a quality of life that I had earned and to which I had every right.

The day of that commitment—January 29, 1993—is the day I served notice to the world, and to myself, that I would not accept being defined by my arthritis. It was a moment of genuine self-liberation.

Once having agreed to go ahead, my first question to Dr. Wolf was: "How soon can we do it?" One phone call later, we had a date I'll never forget: March 15, 1993.

Even as I write these words, almost four years later to the day, I can recall the sense of empowerment I had been missing for the previous several years. I was a different person—or rather, I should say, more like my old self than I had been in a while. I would not be someone to whom things happen but—as I used to be—one of those who make things happen.

Almost immediately my new attitude asserted itself. As the preop period began, I realized I was not *waiting* for surgery but actively *preparing* for it. In fact, I was no longer in the grip of a fraught concept such as "surgery." Instead I was focused on a positive, forward-looking concept: a new knee!

The Science (and Art) of Joint Replacements

When Dr. Wolf first told me I needed a total knee replacement, my first reaction was, "Hey, wait a minute!" After all, if you're talking about replacing a body part, "total" sounds pretty . . . well, total! And the picture that flashed through my mind was something like a heart or liver or kidney transplant. Suddenly I had this completely irrational vision of the middle of my leg being "totally" removed and "totally" replaced by some kind of artificial contraption that would then be my knee for the rest of my life. Later on I learned that my reaction was far from unique. In fact, a total knee replacement—although hardly a piece of cake—is not as drastic as it sounds. As Dr. Wolf points out:

The term "total knee replacement" is a misnomer. The more correct term would be total knee arthroplasty. The suffix -*plasty* means to reconstruct or repair. A total knee arthroplasty reconstructs an arthritic knee by replacing the articular surfaces while preserving the ligaments, tendons, and muscles that are essential to knee function.

The first thing to know about joint replacement is that it is a very young science. The father of modern-day joint replacement was Sir John Charnley, a British orthopedic surgeon who, in the early 1960s, developed and began using the first successful hip prosthesis. Previous prostheses proved unable to withstand the physical impact of everyday life, but Charnley's prosthesis was made of synthetic, high-density polyethylene that could absorb the shock and friction of the metal head. Charnley also secured the prosthesis with methylmetharcrylate cement, a dental glue.

Charnley's prosthesis was a major breakthrough. Not only did it provide relief for his patients. It unleashed a flood of competing total-hip designs. The medical industry invested heavily in the research and development of new and improved designs. Shortly thereafter, prostheses were developed for knees and other joints, and within ten years, the total knee was an effective and practical reality.

Although cement was critical in the performance of the first total hip and knee replacements, its use was not without problems. Some people have a chemical reaction to the cement that can produce a dramatic drop in blood pressure. Cement also ages and becomes brittle and prone to failure after several years. The cement can also crack under repeated stresses and strains, causing the prosthesis to loosen or even break. But, as Dr. Wolf points out:

> While most of these problems were eliminated or minimized by new cement techniques which had been developed by the early eighties, one major unresolved problem remained. This arises when, as a result of instability in a post-operative knee or hip, one or more of the components may have to be revised. Some early revisions are due to technical errors; others because of infection where it is imperative that the prosthesis and the cement be removed to get the infection under control; or a prosthetic compo-

nent can be malpositioned, causing instability of the joint. In such cases, the immediate solidity that cement provides can be a double-edged sword since the need to remove the cement presents serious technical obstacles that can lead to major intra-operative complications.

Consequently, while one school of surgeons was working on improving the cement and the techniques to use it, other surgeons kept looking for alternatives to cement. In the 1970s a new technique was developed in which the bone grows to the surface of the prosthesis and cement is not needed. That's what Dr. Wolf used in all three of my joint replacements. (Actually, a certain amount of cement was used in the knee replacements, not on the femoral and tibial components but only to secure the kneecap.)

As a result, when a noncemented, biologic ingrowth prosthesis requires early revision, the procedure is not as difficult.

Although there have been major improvements in prosthesis design and use of materials, a state-of-the-art joint replacement today is still largely based on Charnley's model. The procedure still consists of reshaping the surfaces of the joint's bony structures to prepare the joint for the insertion of a prosthesis that will be able to do the work a healthy joint does. The prosthesis will probably be made of a combination of metal and plastic materials. The word *total* means that *all* the articulated, cartilage-covered bony structures in a joint will be resurfaced.

In those cases where only one compartment of the knee is affected, it is possible to replace only that part and preserve the rest of the knee. This is called a unicompartmental arthroplasty. This type of "partial replacement" has a much faster recovery and a better functional result, but oddly enough—

according to Dr. Wolf—it is technically more difficult and is performed less frequently than total knee arthroplasty.

On the other hand, the term "total hip replacement" is less of a misnomer because the diseased hip joint is actually resected and totally replaced. And although a total hip replacement is major surgery, the procedure is somewhat less technically demanding than a total knee replacement on what would be considered an equal level of arthritic disease since the hip is inherently more stable and depends less on ligaments for its stability.

In chapter 2, we noted that the hip consists of two components: a ball and a socket. The ball is at the upper end of the femur (the thigh bone), and the socket is at the lower end of the pelvic bone. In a total hip replacement, says Dr. Wolf:

> The orthopedic surgeon will remove the ball and the socket and shape the two bones in order to prepare them for accepting the prosthesis. To do this, a socket will be shaped in the femur into which the stem of the femoral component will be fit. The patient's diseased cup is prepared and reshaped to accept a porous coated metallic cup that has [a] plastic (high-density polyethylene) liner into which the ball of the femoral component will fit.
>
> A total knee replacement is somewhat more complicated because the knee has three bony components—the lower end of the femur (thigh bone), the upper end of the tibia (shin bone) and the patella (kneecap). Unlike the hip, which does not depend on ligaments for its stability, a knee has multiple and essential ligamentous restraints. Without these, the knee would not be stable.
>
> In a total hip replacement, we often sacrifice all the ligamental structures around the hip. If we did that in the knee joint, it would be a disaster. This is what makes a knee

replacement a more complex operation. If you remove the ligaments and replace the surfaces of the knee there's no stability. So in a knee replacement, you have to work with and need to preserve all the tissues—ligaments, muscles, and tendons—around the knee.

Nevertheless, surgeon experience and improved instrumentation have made a primary total knee replacement a relatively standardized procedure.

Instrumentation has been developed to allow exacting cuts with a saw blade to remove the diseased surfaces and shape them to accommodate the components. This is somewhat analogous to shaping a diseased tooth to accept a crown. Then you resurface the kneecap with an all-polyethylene plastic component or a metal-and-polyethylene combination. These components are either press-fit (biologic ingrowth) or cemented into place.

As the demand for joint replacements continues to grow and increasingly involves younger and more physically active patients, surgeons continue to do both cemented and cementless joint replacements. To a great extent, the choice depends on the age and overall physical condition of the patient. Like many other surgeons, Dr. Wolf tends to favor cemented implants for his older, more sedentary patients. Apparently, the recovery time is faster for them since the cement hardens immediately. That allows full weight-bearing activity immediately after surgery. Refinements in the cement have also helped overcome some of the earlier problems. But since cement still has a tendency to age and become brittle, Dr. Wolf believes younger and more active patients are better treated with the biologically fixed (uncemented) prostheses, especially if they plan to get back to a relatively vigorous lifestyle.

Your new joint should enable you to regain most of the functions of a normal joint. It should eliminate most of the pain you felt before, increase your mobility, and, in general, be a big improvement over what you had prior to the replacement. But it will never be the same or as good as a healthy natural joint. You will probably always feel some stiffness in your knees and still have some limitations on your activity. But the main thing is that, by its very nature, a prosthesis is finite. If you are active and live long enough, the best of all prostheses may wear out and have to be replaced.

Two Knees at Once

When Dr. Wolf first recommended that I have a knee replacement, he told me that I would need to have the other knee replaced pretty soon as well and that I also had at least one hip replacement (possibly two) in my future. I wasn't completely surprised since I'd already had arthroscopic surgery on both knees, but the prospect of having both knees and both hips replaced was sobering. The image that popped into my head was that of Boris Karloff as Frankenstein's monster, walking stiff-jointed through the countryside.

Since I'd heard that some people had both knees replaced at the same time, I asked Dr. Wolf whether that was an option for me and what were the pluses and minuses of doing both at once. He said:

> I've done two knees at once many times. The pluses are that you get it over with. It saves an operative event. You combine the two events into one anesthetic. It's one hospi-

tal stay instead of two, although you'll be in the hospital longer than with just one knee.

The minuses are that you have an increased level of postoperative pain. It's more of a shock to the system, and it's a longer recovery. If you have two knees done at the same time, then you may need to have more blood on hand, more transfusions. The more transfusions you have, the greater the risks of complications related to transfusions. And while the anesthetic event is reduced to one instead of two, it's a longer anesthetic, and if you looked at the statistics, you'd probably find that the longer the time under an anesthetic, the more likely a complication will arise from the procedure.

On the other hand, if both knees are equally bad and you're unable to distinguish one being the problem knee and the other being tolerable—then it's probably better to do both knees at once. And then you have some people who have personal time considerations—maybe they don't want to take that much time off from work twice—and they just want to get it all done at once and not come back.

In my case, Dr. Wolf's judgment was that there was enough of a difference between my two knees so that I would probably be better off having them replaced one at a time. It was a good call. By the time I absolutely needed to have my other knee replaced, eight months later, I had pretty well recovered from the first operation. Consequently, my first knee was able to support me when I had the second one done.

My physical therapist, Karen Sandy, has treated double-knee-replacement patients but doesn't recommend the procedure.

I think it's much better to wait. Most doctors will ask you which one hurts the worst; then when you recover from

the first, you've got at least one good, strong, pain-free leg.
And that usually helps the recovery on the second one.
Usually it will be faster.

One of my E-mail correspondents, who calls herself Lady
Andy, found another solution. She has psoriatic arthritis,
which resulted in severe contractures in both knees. (A con-
tracture is a stiffening of the joint that limits—or even prevents—bending and curtails range of motion.) A double
surgery seemed to be called for since the damage to both legs
was so extreme she would have had great difficulty walking
after just one. Rather than replacing both knees at once, however, her surgeon recommended doing them one after
another with a two-week interval. Then forty-seven, Lady
Andy had the first knee done January 10, 1997, but delayed
the second for an additional two weeks, until February 11,
1997. Both surgeries were performed by Dr. Clive M. Segil at
the Cedars-Sinai Medical Center in Los Angeles. In both
cases, she spent four days in the hospital and another four
days in a skilled nursing facility.

Two weeks after the second knee replacement, Lady Andy
wrote: "I'm beginning to use crutches instead of the walker. I'm
able to drive on my own and only need occasional pain medicine
before physical therapy. One thing I'm particularly happy
with is how my first knee has served me during this period with
the second one. It is able to hold my full weight without any
problem or pain, and it still isn't fully recovered itself."

The Risks

Part of being fully informed about a joint replacement is knowing the risks. One of the things that gave me confidence in Dr. Wolf was that he didn't mince any words in telling me about them.

One of the risks of surgery, even though you may not have any cardiac problems, or diabetes or high blood pressure or any other particular risk factors, is death. It is a very small risk, but it does exist, especially when you operate on relatively aged, sometimes fragile people who have some medical problems. So I always make sure they know the risks of surgery and what the operation is all about. I tell them, "We've tried nonoperative care for an extended period and your arthritis has progressed. We've tried medicines, injections, and perhaps even arthroscopic surgery, but they have lost their effectiveness." Of course, the final decision is the patient's. I just want to make sure they understand the risks.

One of the biggest concerns in joint-replacement surgery is the possibility of infection in the new joint. Despite adherence to the most rigorous sterile operating room techniques, bacteria from the patient or from the ambient air can contaminate the wound and infect the prosthesis in the early postoperative period. Late infections can occur from bacteria that travel through the blood from a faraway site in the body. Bacteria that manage to get into the blood seem to have a tendency to adhere to prosthetic devices in the body. The danger can occur when you have a surgical or dental procedure that sends bacteria into the bloodstream—such as going to the dentist for your semiannual cleaning. If those bacteria get into your blood and happen to find your new knee as they travel through your body and decide to stop there, you're in big trouble. Once that knee or prosthesis gets infected the chances of salvaging it are 50-50.

This is why joint-replacement patients are usually advised to take antibiotics immediately before and after they have dental work or other surgical procedures. (Dr. Susan Hoch recommends taking antibiotics the same way when having a cystoscopy, a sigmoidoscopy, a colonoscopy, or dilation and curettage [D&C].) Unfortunately, people my age find themselves going to the dentist or the periodontist much more often than we did when we were younger. (I have since been told by both Dr. Wolf and my dentist that this practice of medicating with antibiotics is being phased out for most dental procedures.)

According to Dr. Wolf, the statistics show that approximately one joint replacement patient in 300 ever gets some kind of infection. He adds:

If a serious deep infection occurs in your knee, you're in for additional operations to save that prosthesis, and if that fails the prosthesis may have to be removed while the infection is eradicated. Infections can occur early, within the first few weeks following the operation, or late, months or years after the initial procedure. One of my patients got an infection 12 years after her total knee. I did a total shoulder replacement on another patient who postoperatively had a significant intestinal infection—the bowel bacteria seeded and infected her prosthesis and it had to be removed.

Infection can occur in the immediate postoperative period. Despite the fact that everyone in the operating room scrubs their hands, wears gloves and protective clothing, and uses sterile techniques, there is always some risk of contamination of the wound in the operating room itself. For one thing, the air in the operating room is not sterile. So when you open up the body, it's exposed to the air. If you're immunocompromised, or you have poor blood supply or you're a diabetic, there is a higher chance of infection from that contamination. The normal person has defense mechanisms that can eliminate most bacteria that happen into the wound while it's open.

This is what happened to Ron Fowler's sixty-eight-year-old mother. She had her left hip replaced in the summer of 1995 in a hospital in England. When he told me the story a year later, he wrote:

The operation seemed to go OK but she had stomach trouble for a week or so after which prevented her eating much. Then, about three weeks later, an infection showed up in the hip. The doctors treated her with antibiotics but the infection proved resistant and she went back to hospital where they opened up the wound three times to clean it.

After a month in hospital the problem seemed to have cleared up so they let her go home. But the infection returned again and the doctors decided to completely remove the new hip and leave it out for six to eight weeks hoping this would clear it up. But it didn't and after seven weeks, the doctors said she'd have to wait another 2–3 months before they could redo the hip. To make matters worse, her other (right) hip is now going bad. Her doctor's latest suggestion is to replace the right hip while still leaving the left hip alone for the moment. This sounds a bit risky to me since, if the infection then turns up in the new replacement, things would be very unpleasant.

Fortunately, Ron's story has a happy ending. In March 1997, he wrote: "My mother now has two working hips. She had the previously infected hip replaced about three weeks ago."

I asked Dr. Wolf to explain the procedure used to treat an infected joint:

> The first thing you do, of course, is wash it out. You try to clean it without removing the components. We clean and debride all infected tissues, place drains, and give you appropriate antibiotics to stop the infection. As is the case with all infection, if you catch it early, clean it out early, wash it early, you start the antibiotics early, you get the cultures quickly, the better the chance of stopping it before it becomes a chronic problem. Most of the time you can stop that infection before it involves and destroys the adjacent bone.
>
> Another risk from joint-replacement surgery is the possibility of a blood clot forming in veins deep in your leg. That's why all joint-replacement patients receive some kind of preventive treatment with respect to deep-vein thrombosis. The use of compressive stockings to prevent blood from pooling is almost universal. There are also alternative compression foot pumps and stockings that apply intermittent pressure to the lower extremities via a small electric pump at the bedside. Anticoagulant medications (blood thinners) such as heparin or Coumadin are also used by many surgeons in the immediate postoperative period to prevent deep-vein thrombosis.
>
> But the simplest and least complicated way of preventing clots is through early mobilization of the patient. That means up and out of bed walking on the first postoperative day. In spite of all prophylactic measures, however, there are rare cases where a blood clot forms. This will produce

increased pain and swelling in the involved extremity. An increased dose of anticoagulant medications such as heparin will rapidly dissolve the clot. If left untreated, the clot could travel to your lung, producing what is known as an "embolus." Most emboli are very small and produce no symptoms, but a very large embolus in the lung could be life-threatening.

The most common untoward outcome of a total knee arthroplasty is one where the range of motion of the prosthetic knee is limited. Although some people get what we call arthro-fibrosis, where the knee becomes inflamed and scars down, the most significant predictor of limited motion postoperatively is the preoperative range of motion. Osteoarthritis can lead to progressive deformity and loss of motion. Those patients whose disease has progressed to a point where the range of motion has been lost preoperatively have a much more difficult time regaining a good functional range after surgery. Their ligaments, tendons and muscles can be very difficult to rehabilitate if their arthritis and preoperative deformity are significant. Some people wait too long to decide to proceed with the surgery.

Some people just seem to get stuck. And there's a small minority of patients—in the realm of less than 5 percent—to whom I have to say: "You know what, it's been three months and your progress is a little too slow in regaining your motion. I want to take you back to the operating room and put you under a general anesthetic for a few minutes. I will manipulate your knee and break down the scar that is preventing you from moving your knee." This usually accelerates the patient's recovery and the range of motion is improved.

Another thing to keep in mind is that people have different levels of pain tolerance. Dr. Wolf tells of a patient who went into surgery with what he describes as "the most horrible deformed knee."

I was sure that he would have severe postoperative pain. Well, he woke up and—no pain. This man had undergone an extensive surgery. Still, on the first day after surgery when I went into his room, he said, "Thank you, Doctor. Thank you!" If someone has been in pain for months or even years, they tend to develop increased tolerance for pain. This man had been in great pain for several years and he had a very difficult situation. Patients who are truly experiencing a lot of pain are much more willing to accept the surgical pain and endure the difficulties of the postoperative period. Someone who has marginal symptomatology is more likely to have a problem with the postoperative pain.

Anesthesia

Many people facing surgery have more anxiety about the anesthesia than they do about the surgery itself. I'm like that. Many years ago I had "minor surgery" for a hernia that was performed with spinal anesthesia. That's when I learned that "minor surgery" is defined as surgery that happens to someone else. For me, there was nothing "minor" about it. Because I was more or less awake during the operation, I found myself growing increasingly tense as the surgery proceeded. And when it was over, I hated the feeling of helplessness generated by the lack of sensation in the lower half of my body as I waited for the anesthesia to wear off.

On the other hand, I also hate the idea of losing consciousness and "going under." That probably means I'm a bit of a control freak, but I bet a lot of people feel the same way. Nevertheless, if you're going to have surgery, who among us would be willing to forgo the anesthesia? (Years ago, on a visit to China, I witnessed a major operation in which the patient was fully awake while acupuncture successfully served the function of the anesthesia.)

The choice of anesthesia is one of the decisions you will be asked to make when having a joint replacement. In general, the choice is between general anesthesia and an epidural (a local anesthetic, injected near the spinal cord, that numbs the lower half of your body). Pretty much at the urging of the surgeons, I've had general anesthesia with all six of my joint-related surgeries—three knee arthroscopies and three joint replacements.

Dr. Wolf said there were pros and cons to both and that the risk was pretty much the same for each. But it was obvious that he was pushing me to go the general anesthesia route. Here is what he says:

> One of the things about epidural anesthetics is that they're not 100 percent effective. Sometimes you run into problems and you then have to go to a general. That not only wastes a lot of time, but it can be uncomfortable for the patient.
>
> I had one patient who asked for an epidural because he wanted to watch the operation. He couldn't watch continuously, but at a certain point he wanted to see where we were. And at each point we would position him so that he could look over the sheets and look down at his knee. He was actually very calm about it, very matter-of-fact.

One reassuring note: Citing experts who estimate "it's safer to have general anesthesia than to ride in a car," the

Mayo Clinic says that "anesthesia is ten times safer than it was in the 1970s and 100 times safer than it was in 1955. Fast-acting medications, new monitoring devices plus higher safety standards for their use are credited with reducing complications and accidental deaths during general anesthesia." (*Mayo Clinic Health Letter*, March 1995)

Preop Blood Donation

As soon as my surgery date was settled, Dr. Wolf told me I would have to arrange to have three pints of my own blood available for use in the operating room during surgery. The idea behind this, he said, was that "when you lose blood during surgery we replace it with your own blood. That makes it totally safe. You can't catch anything from yourself."

Or, to put it another way, it's like masturbation—the ultimate safe sex.

If you're in an HMO, there is probably a procedure for this purpose in place. Otherwise, the easiest way to do this is through the Red Cross, which has blood donation services just about everywhere. The Red Cross doesn't want to take more than one pint of blood from you at a time, so I had to schedule three visits. The time frame for giving blood is important: The first donation no more than six weeks before the operation and the last no sooner than two weeks before. Dr. Wolf gave me an authorization slip with all the necessary information concerning my surgery so that the donations could be scheduled appropriately and the Red Cross would know when and where to deliver the blood. However, since the blood is going for your own surgery, it's not exactly a donation, so you're likely to be charged for it. It cost me $20 for each pint.

You should not donate blood if you've got a cold or the flu or an infection since these conditions will compromise the blood you'll get back during surgery. (You'll be reminded of this just before you give blood.) You should eat a nourishing meal two to four hours prior to your blood donation. And no strenuous exercise until the next day.

Most of us get a little anxious about giving blood. In fact, both your blood and your blood consistency will be measured before your blood is taken. It's not uncommon for people to have an elevated blood pressure level just before giving blood. That usually indicates some anxiety. In such cases, the nurses have you rest quietly, give you some juice, and wait until your blood pressure goes down before going ahead. Similarly, if your blood demonstrates some level of anemia you might be advised to take an iron supplement or—contrary to the way you might usually eat—to go heavy on the red meat. Some people have even been known to faint after giving blood—whether from a sudden drop in blood pressure or because of a nervous reaction to seeing their own blood in the plastic bag. Not to worry. The nurses have seen it all and know what to do.

In addition to the obvious benefits to using your own blood in the age of AIDS, there's a psychological plus, too. The very process of giving blood is good mental preparation for the surgery. It helps take you out of the passive mode of having something done to you and conditions you to being an active participant in the process of getting your new knee or hip.

Handicapped Parking

One thing you can do—if you haven't already—is apply for a handicapped-parking placard. These are absolute lifesavers, and if you're ready for a joint replacement, you're undoubtedly ready and qualified for one. Regulations vary from state to state, but in California these permit you not only to park in designated handicapped spaces but to park indefinitely and without feeding the meter at any metered space. You can also park indefinitely at any unmetered, limited-parking space. They are also reciprocally honored in every state in the United States.

And they're not hard to get. You just get a form from the Department of Motor Vehicles (DMV) and ask your doctor to fill it out and sign it. When you bring it back to the DMV, approval is virtually automatic. (Of course, if you've faked the doctor's signature, that's a crime and you place yourself in peril of legal prosecution.) You don't even have to be a driver to get one. Anyone who is acting as your chauffeur can use it *while you are a passenger.*

In California, there are two types of handicapped-parking permits: temporary (six months) and permanent (two years with no doctor's signature required for renewal). Both cost $6.

Your general health is an important factor in ensuring a successful operation and a problem-free recovery. If you're a smoker, try to stop during the preop period. Not only will this help get your body to maximum health for the surgery, it might get you on the track to quitting altogether. And if ever there was a time for a balanced, sensible diet—low fat, high fiber, no junk food, lots of fruit and vegetables—this is it. You also might want to consider vitamin supplements during this period. The Arthritis Foundation suggests: "Vitamin C may enhance the healing process after surgery."

Preop Exercises

One of the best things you can do in preparation for a joint replacement is exercise. Of course, by the time you make a decision to have a knee or a hip replaced, you're usually having so much pain that the idea of exercise during the preop period might seem ridiculous. As a result, many people simply reduce their activity to a bare minimum and basically wait for the surgeon.

Big mistake—especially if you have osteoarthritis. (Given the nature of their disease, rheumatoid arthritis patients who have gotten to the point of surgery might have a harder time exercising in the preop period. But even then, every effort should be made to find some type of physical activity you can handle.)

You should be looking for three types of exercise: aerobic (or endurance) exercises, which serve to strengthen your cardiovascular system; exercises that will strengthen the muscles in the vicinity of the affected joint; and range-of-motion exercises, in which you move your joints as far as possible.

Clearly you're going to be looking for exercise that is not weight-bearing. So don't even think about jogging or tennis— let alone racquetball or basketball. In fact, it's probably safe to say that most competitive sports are off the list. For people like myself that's a big adjustment. My social conditioning growing up was that all sports—with a few exceptions such as bike riding and hiking—were competitive.

In terms of aerobic exercises, I focused on two: bike riding and swimming. Actually, as I mentioned earlier, I had been doing both ever since I was forced to stop playing tennis—so, for me, it was more a matter of making sure I kept them up.

The bike riding was quite pleasurable, although after a while I began to feel insecure—even on bike paths—about having to cope with other cyclists, pedestrians, folks pushing baby carriages, potholes, and the like. I finally switched to an exercise bike at home. Not as much fun, but I set it up in front of the TV and watched old movies on my VCR.

I did feel some hip pain while swimming, although it wasn't bad enough that I had to stop. But even if you don't or can't swim, water exercises can be very helpful.

Maryanne Kufs of Adams, Massachusetts, has been a resource teacher for preschool children for more than twenty-five years. "You'd be surprised," she writes, "at how many preschool teachers and providers of day care have arthritis. In a class with small children you are up and down from floor to standing, you are sitting in very small chairs, you are picking children up, stepping over and around them." Maryanne has had two hip replacements due to severe osteoarthritis, the first in 1986 and the second in 1997, both done at St. Peter's Hospital in Albany, New York, by Dr. Carl Wirth. She writes:

> I would urge hip-replacement patients to work out in the water both as preparation for a hip replacement and as part of the rehab therapy after surgery. In preparation for my second hip replacement, I began working out in the water at the local Holiday Inn eight months earlier. By the time of my surgery, I had improved my bone density and created a strong muscle base as well as better general health. I also did water therapy after the surgery. I believe these workouts were the primary factor in my quick rehabilitation and return to normal life. It's not "just swimming" and it's not exactly water aerobics but it provides a good aerobic, muscle-building, and fat-burning workout that is as diverse as the person who creates it. It has changed my life!

A few months into my preop pool workouts, I found a great book that had all the exercises I was doing and more, as well as sections for hip- and knee-replacement patients. It's called *The Complete Waterpower Workout Book: Programs for Fitness, Injury Prevention, and Healing,* by Lynda Huey, Robert Forster, and Pete Romano (New York: Random House, 1993).

According to *Consumer Reports on Health:*

Simple exercises to promote flexibility and strengthen the muscles around the knee can go a long way toward warding off problems. In many cases, they can also help hasten recovery after knee injury or surgery. The three basic exercises shown here, suggested by the Arthritis Foundation, can be especially helpful.

For maximum benefit, perform the exercises once or twice a day, repeating each one 5 to 10 times for each knee. If you already have knee pain, check with your doctor or physical therapist to see if these exercises should be adapted to your particular problem.

Preparing Your Home

Presurgery is the time to start preparing your home for what you will need after you get home from the hospital. My situation was pretty good that way. My wife, who is a singer, was able to be at home with me most of the time. And we were living in a single-level apartment in a building with an elevator, so I was able to function without having to navigate stairs at all.

But if there are stairs in your home, and you're going to

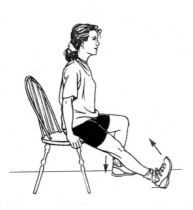

THIGH FIRMER

Sit on the edge of a chair with one leg stretched out in front and the heel resting on the floor. Tighten the muscle that runs across the front of the knee by flexing your toes back. At the same time, push the back of the knee down toward the floor until you feel a stretch there as well as at the back of the ankle. Hold for five seconds.

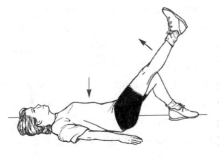

STRAIGHT LEG LIFT

Lie on your back with one knee bent and the foot flat on the floor. Keep your stomach pulled in and your back flat. Extend the other leg and lift it slowly as far as you comfortably can without bending that knee. Hold for five seconds and slowly lower the leg. (Note: don't do this exercise if you have hip pain.)

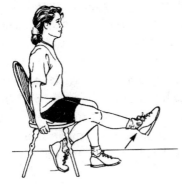

KNEE FLEXION
AND EXTENSION

Bend your knee by pulling your heel under the chair and hold for about five seconds. Keeping your foot relaxed, slowly raise it up to straighten the knee. Hold for another five seconds and then slowly lower your foot to the floor.

have long stretches where you'll be on your own, you might want to set up a temporary living space for yourself on one floor—one with both a bathroom and a kitchen.

Check out potential hazards in your home. Remember, you're going to be getting around with a walker or crutches for a while when you get back. So get rid of clutter, making sure you have wide, clear passageways. Remove any throw rugs and tape down electrical cords that present a potential tripping risk.

If you have stairs, make sure you have a banister. If you already have handrails, check to make sure they're strong and secure. Even if you have just a couple of steps at the entrance to your home, make sure you have something secure to grab on to when you're using them.

Put items you use often within easy reach—preferably between waist and shoulder level. You won't want to be bending or reaching (especially with a hip replacement), and you definitely do not want to be getting on footstools.

If you live alone or will be spending periods when you are on your own, stock up on canned and frozen foods. Here's when a microwave oven can be pretty helpful. You might also want to look into services such as Meals on Wheels that deliver meals. Find out what services your city and/or county government offers. Most localities have some kind of organization in charge of senior citizens' services (in Oakland it's listed under the Department of Adult and Aging Services) and a social services agency. Unless they've since been wiped out by budget cuts, you'll be amazed at the kinds of help that can be provided.

Postop seating is something you don't want to have to start thinking about after you come home from the hospital. What you will find is that most of your favorite sitting places are too low. (Again, this is especially important if you've had a hip replacement.) The American Academy of Orthopedic Surgeons recommends: "A stable chair with a firm seat cushion (18–20 inches in height), a firm back, two arms, and a footstool for intermittent leg elevation." This will enable you to sit up straight, and the armrests will provide additional leverage when you're getting up. And avoid sitting for extended periods. When you're watching TV, get up and walk around a bit during commercial breaks. You won't miss much.

If, like me, you have a favorite recliner, you'll probably need to elevate it. I had a special riser attached to the bottom of mine. Couches might look inviting, but they are next to impossible to get out of. Four years after my hip replacement I still avoid sitting on a couch unless it's higher than average and there's a firm armrest in easy reach. Even then, it's always something of an adventure.

The same thing applies to your bed. I was fortunate in that we already had a twenty-two-inch-high queen-size platform bed with a good, firm mattress. But if your bed is in the more typical sixteen-inches-high range, you should probably figure out a way to elevate it to at least eighteen inches. And get a bed board or an extrafirm mattress.

It's also a good idea to have a firm pillow to sit on when you're in a car.

Special Equipment

There's a wide assortment of special equipment you might find useful even in the preop period.

Getting in and out of a bathtub is the most dangerous thing you'll do at home after your surgery. So, if you have to use a tub—even if it's just for the shower—have grab bars installed. Even if you have a walk-in shower, you'll probably want something strong to hold on to as you go in and out. A physical therapist can give you the best advice on where these should be located. You'll also want a stable shower bench or chair for bathing.

Almost everyone I know who has had a joint replacement has used an elevated toilet seat. I did. Without it, I might still be sitting there. Get one with arms to give you leverage when you sit down and get up.

If you're ready for a joint replacement, you're probably already using a cane. I had never used one before—except for an occasional display of jauntiness—so I thought any cane would do. Not so. The height of your cane is crucial. According to Karen, "When you stand straight with your hands at your side, the top of the cane should come to your wrist bone." Your best bet is a lightweight, adjustable metal cane. (Some of them also fold, which can be a convenience.)

There are also lots of techniques for moving things—dollies, slides, straps—other than straight lifting. But don't be embarrassed about asking for help when you need to lift something heavy or bulky. And if it's too uncomfortable, get someone else to do it. Remember, people want to help—especially when they see you doing everything you can to help yourself.

Preop Classes

Some people awaiting surgery want to know everything they can about it, including what's going to take place in the operating room. Others try not to think about it until the last minute, although that rarely prevents them from worrying. The fact is, however, that the more you know, the better off you are.

According to *Consumer Reports on Health* (August 1997),

"All preparatory measures, whether physical or mental, generate a sense of involvement and control that may not only calm your mind but actually speed your recovery. . . . An analysis of the combined results of 68 studies found that knowing what to expect before, during and after surgery not only allayed apprehension but also improved overall recovery by an average of 20 percent." (Back issues of *Consumer Reports on Health* are available for just $3. Write them at 101 Truman Avenue, Yonkers, New York 10703-1057.)

Dr. Wolf is a wonderful guy and a great surgeon. If it turns out I need to have my other hip replaced, I'll go back to him. But I must say that he didn't prepare me for dealing with all of the difficulties and details I encountered in my first postop situation. I've heard the same thing from other joint-replacement patients.

Hospitals should take more responsibility for patient preparation. When I had my joint replacements done I didn't even know that some hospitals offered preop classes. Fortunately, that situation is beginning to change. More and more hospitals are now assuming the responsibility for preop instruction for their joint-replacement patients. This might be one area where HMOs will do better than Medicare, since it has been proven that preop instruction actually saves hospital time and can speed up recovery time.

Among the facilities I know of that now offer preop instruction classes to joint-replacement patients are the Kaiser Hospitals in California, the Hospital for Special Surgery in New York City, and the University of Iowa Hospitals and Clinics. There must be others as well. I sat in on the hip-replacement class at Kaiser, which covered everything from the moment you check into the hospital through a detailed account of the surgery and inpatient recovery process to the mechanics of your discharge and transportation home. It also included crutch and walker training.

The Hospital for Special Surgery (HSS), which concentrates on orthopedic and rheumatologic conditions, provides joint-replacement patients with an excellent, detailed book, *Your Pathway to Recovery*, one for knees and one for hips.

Kaiser offers a calendar advising patients what to do and what to expect from four to six weeks prior to surgery until six weeks after surgery. Iowa has a similar calendar plus an informational pamphlet.

The Doctors' Medical Center in Pinole, California, has taken the idea of preop classes for joint-replacement patients one step further. They have initiated what they call their Joint Works Special Program. Directed by Patty Donahue, an RN with twenty-five years' experience in the field of oryhopedics, the program assembles a group of knee- and hip-replacement patients who will go through the experience together—from a joint preop class to in-hospital postop therapy and exercises.

The group is kept together in the same section of the hospital and gathers regularly in a special room put aside for their use. Once they can get out of bed, they take their meals together. All this socialization enables them to exchange experiences with one another and to offer one another psychological support.

The Center has found, says Donahue, that "patients who go through this program together find they have less fear because they are not going through the experience alone, and they actually have less pain."

Many of the groups stay in touch with one another after they leave the hospital. Several have developed a tradition of annual Christmas parties together.

The program apparently originated with the Florida Knee & Hip Clinic in Clearwater and has been taken up by more than twenty-five hospitals nationwide. (Hospitals interested in looking into the program can reach the Clinic's Orthopedic Marketing System at 800-741-3877.)

If your hospital does not offer a preop class or a written guide for patients, ask your surgeon to tell you in detail what's going to happen on the day of surgery, what kind of anesthesia will be used, and so forth. Ask him to show you a model of the prosthesis you're going to get. Some people might not want to know all the details of what goes on in the operating room, but I found that having a sense of the procedure and the medical technology was very reassuring.

Also ask him what you can expect after the operation. It's a little unsettling when a nurse suddenly shows up and starts inserting a tube into your body. Unless you've been told beforehand that this is standard procedure, you might think that an unexpected problem has come up. And ask about anything else that crosses your mind. When do you start eating again? How often and when will your surgeon be visiting you? What kind of pain can you anticipate and what measures will be taken to keep you comfortable?

One thing I'd especially urge: Ask your surgeon to prescribe a home preop visit by a physical therapist. My physical therapist, Karen Sandy, who has helped rehabilitate thousands of joint-replacement patients, says:

It would make this whole procedure so much better if everybody having joint-replacement surgery were evaluated by a physical therapist beforehand. They could be taught isometric exercises to try to build up their gluteal and quad strength and get their leg as strong as possible. And it's always an advantage to teach someone exercises before surgery. That way they learn the exercises, they know what to expect, and they know what their muscles felt like when they were doing them before surgery.

It would also give us an idea of what that person is like beforehand, what their personality is. This is very useful information for us. We can also reassure them if they're worried.

A physical therapist can also help you decide whether you want to use crutches or a walker when you come home from the hospital. This is a decision better made before rather than after surgery so that you can get some preliminary training. In general, Karen prefers a walker, which is what I used.

The only reason to use crutches is if you have to navigate stairs. And if you're younger and you want to go much faster, although we don't like people rushing around. Those are the only advantages of crutches. I think initially a walker is much better. It gives you more stability. You don't have to worry about a walker falling over or dropping.

Medical Preparations

Finally, there are important medical preparations you will have to make. For one thing, you should see your primary care doctor a few days before the operation. If you don't, the hospital itself will give you a complete physical checkup, which will probably include an electro-cardiogram. But it's better to have your own doctor, who is familiar with your medical history and your medications, do it.

Make sure your surgeon is aware of all the medications you take—both prescription and over-the-counter. Some medicines don't mix well with anesthesia. Others, such as NSAIDs (including ibuprofen), aspirin, and blood thinners increase bleeding. Also make sure your doctor knows whether you are allergic to any medicines. If you are allergic to penicillin, as I am, it's important that your surgeon know this beforehand, especially since certain antibiotics that might be prescribed for you have a penicillin base.

It's also a good idea to get any pending dental work completed before your operation. If you have bleeding gums or are expecting to have a tooth pulled, or if you are in the midst of root-canal work—get it done. Otherwise, as previously mentioned, bacteria in the mouth could enter the bloodstream and cause an infection in the area of the replacement or in the new joint itself. And wait several weeks after surgery before getting a cleaning or any other dental work.

Showtime

inally, the Big Day arrives. You've done everything you can. You've given blood. You've done your preop exercises, and you've been to a preop class. You've gotten your home prepared for when you come back from the hospital. Now it's up to the surgeon and the rest of the operating room crew.

Just remember: This is the Big Day not because you're having surgery, although you can't help but think about that. The truly big thing is that today's the day you're going to get your new knee or hip. It's a new beginning. It really is the first day of the rest of your life.

The Day Before

s with any major elective operation, the Big Day actually begins when you go to the hospital a day or two before to preregister. You'll get a round of preop testing—EKG, blood pressure, signs of infection, and so on—if you haven't already had this done by your own physician. I've done this three times and it always felt a little strange to be doing it on my own, since you usually associate "hospital" and "major surgery" with a condition signifying that if you're not at death's door, you're at least pretty sick. Actually, these were useful reminders that I was a basically healthy person capable of looking after myself—or I would be once I had my new knee or hip.

Then there's the night before the operation, when you've been told not to have anything to eat or drink after midnight. This is to make sure there's nothing in your stomach while you're under anesthesia—the danger being that the anesthesia could provoke vomiting, which could choke off your oxygen supply while you are undergoing surgery. (Remember the movie *The Verdict*, with Paul Newman as the alcoholic lawyer suing a hospital on behalf of a patient who had eaten just an hour before having emergency surgery? The doctor had not bothered to check the admitting chart to see when she had last eaten.) Even if you're going to have an epidural (spinal) rather than a general anesthetic, this rule must be followed since there is always the possibility that the epidural won't work and a general will have to be administered instead.

It's a good idea to leave your valuables (watch, wallet, jewelry) at home. But bring your glasses, hearing aid, and dentures. (Put these in plastic bags or containers with your name and hospital registration number.) Also, bring along a book or two. I also carried a few dollars just in case and was always able to find someone willing to buy a copy of the *New York Times* for me. And wear loose clothing. That's what you'll be wearing when you go home and it will have to go over a bulky bandage or dressing.

All three of my joint replacements were done on Monday, which is good for two reasons. First, you can usually leave the hospital by Friday and not have to spend the weekend in a hospital bed for an extra couple of days when they won't be doing much for you anyway. (The in-house physical therapist doesn't work on weekends.) And second, I like to believe that a surgeon is feeling at his best after the weekend.

Anyway, since I was the first surgery on Dr. Wolf's schedule, at 7:30 A.M., I was in bed long before midnight. (Some hospitals will admit you the afternoon before, but in these cost-cutting times, most joint-replacement patients go into the hospital on the same day their surgery is scheduled to take place.) I had to be at the hospital at 6:00 A.M. I think the theory behind this is why get everyone all revved up for the operation until you're absolutely certain the star is on hand. So I was up at five, which was a lot harder on my wife (who is a night person) than for me (I usually have half a day's work done by the time she turns over).

Even then, driving over the Bay Bridge from Oakland to San Francisco at 5:30 in the morning, I was amazed how many people are already up and in their cars. Did they all have surgery dates?

At the Hospital

As we drove, I kept telling myself over and over again, "Remember, this is the road to Wellville." And by the time I got to the hospital, all I could think about was that the months of pain and frustration would soon be over. When I was shown to a dressing room where I would change into a hospital gown, I told the nurse, "You've never seen anyone looking forward to surgery as much as I am." I thought that was pretty brave of me then. Later on, I found out that nurses handling joint-replacement patients hear that all the time.

As instructed—it's remarkable how docile you tend to get when dealing with the hospital bureaucracy, as though a failure to follow even the most minute instruction can have dire consequences—we got to the hospital at six. When I checked in at the registration desk and saw my name on the bulletin board for the day's surgeries, the whole affair began to take on a somewhat surreal quality for me. Was I really about to turn my body over to these folks? I kept telling myself, Don't worry, they've done hundreds—probably thousands—of these operations. Yeah, said my other self, but there's always a first time. Well, you can't turn back now, I replied, which brought that conversation to an end.

The precise routine at this point undoubtedly varies from one hospital to another, but basically a small army of nurses, orderlies, interns, and then your impact players—the surgeon and his crew, the anesthesiologist, the RNs—take over.

The first thing they do is put a plastic band with your name and a hospital number on your wrist. This supposedly means you've become hospital "property." Mostly, I guess, it's to make sure they're operating on the right person. Also, they don't want to lose you in some rarely used hospital corridor. The band will also indicate an allergy warning. (Mine was a special color indicating I was allergic to penicillin.) You'll wear this until you're discharged.

From then on until you're out of surgery and in your own room at the hospital, you'll be pretty much in passive mode. Things will be done to and for you, but there's nothing much for you to do except take off your clothes and get into a hospital gown.

A nurse will come around to hook up an IV (intravenous) drip in the back of your hand. This is the way you will get fluids, medication, the anesthesia, and later on, food. She will also take your blood pressure. Get used to that one. It will be done another three or four times before you even get into the operating room and another couple of times in the operating room. You'll also have your temperature taken. That's to make sure you don't have some slight infection, which is a big no-no in surgery. For the same reason, an antibiotic will probably be slipped into your IV.

The only real surprise came when one of the attending nurses put tight-fitting surgical stockings on both my legs. These are compression stockings designed to keep pressure on your legs from your toes up to your thighs. They're called antiembolism and antithrombosis prophylaxis, and they're used to prevent blood clots from forming in your legs. Clots can occur because after the anesthesia wears off you're in pain—which is normal—and you're not going to move the leg very much. The pressure from the stocking keeps blood from pooling in your veins.

You'll also be given a pair of nonskid socks in case you need to go off to the bathroom prior to surgery, which, more than likely, you will.

And then, at some point, the anesthesiologist will visit you. He'll ask you whether or not you've ever had a bad reaction to any particular kind of anesthesia in the past and will explain what type he's planning to use. He'll also answer any questions you might have about the anesthesia.

Finally, it's time for the long ride to the operating room. That's another one of those potentially nerve-racking moments when you might want to remind yourself that millions of people have had the exact same procedure performed with good results. I also found it somewhat reassuring to note how busy the surgery area was. I wasn't the only one having surgery that morning, and realizing that some of the people lying on gurneys nearby were headed for open-heart surgery or removal of a cancerous tumor helped put my own situation into perspective. Anyway, there must have been at least two dozen nurses, orderlies, surgeons, and other doctors busy with various tasks—all of them engendering a climate of confidence-building professionalism.

The only slightly disconcerting note was the number of people who asked me which knee was going to be replaced. Even Dr. Wolf, when he stopped by to say hello, mused aloud, "Let's see. It's the right knee, isn't it?" The attention to this far-from-minor detail would suggest that, however rarely, every once in a while the wrong knee or hip is opened up. After all, stuff happens.

In the Operating Room

After what seemed like an interminable wait—it was really only a few minutes—I was wheeled into the operating room. The OR (as we "veterans" call it) is a place that reeks of technology and sterilization. The first thing that caught my attention was the operating table, sitting there in the middle of the room waiting for me. And no one in the room, except you, has a face. Everyone's wearing a surgical mask, and they're all busy in that cheerfully manic manner that professionals get into as they approach the moment when, for two hours or so, your body will command their undivided attention. As I took all this in, my mind began to flash on all those movies about doctors and operating rooms—I imagined the zigzag lines of the electrocardiogram suddenly going flat or the doctor crisply saying "Scalpel" to the nurse—and despite all my brave thoughts to the contrary I began wondering whether I really should be doing this. But by then, turning back was not an option.

After a while, when I had more or less gotten used to that

scene, I suddenly realized that I was shivering. At first I figured it was just an attack of nerves—mine. But then it dawned on me that it really was cold in there. So the next time a nurse asked me how I was doing, I told her I was cold and in a jiffy I had a bunch of heated blankets on me. After that . . . Dr. Wolf was standing over me saying, "Wake up, Irwin. It's all over!"

Later on, after a series of interviews with Dr. Wolf and an opportunity to sit in on a knee-replacement operation myself, I got a pretty good idea of what goes on in the operating room after they put you out. In general, the procedures for a knee replacement are not much different from those for a hip replacement.

The first thing to know is that it gets pretty crowded in there. There's usually at least six people present at all times.

First, of course, there's the surgeon, who is totally in charge from the beginning of the incision to the last stitch. The operating room, thank goodness, is not a democracy. Nor would any of us lying there on the table want it to be.

The surgeon will also have an assistant in attendance at all times. The assistant may be another surgeon who has elected to spend a year in training with this surgeon, or a postresidency graduate student.

Next is the anesthesiologist, who, in addition to putting you out, also monitors your vital signs throughout the surgery.

Several nurses are also in constant attendance. One works directly with the surgeon. She has to be familiar with the procedure and know the name, shape, size, and appearance of every instrument that will be required in the course of the surgery. Because she has to have the instruments ready even before the doctor asks for them, she has to remember the usual sequence in which they are likely to be called for.

During the operation I sat in on, a representative from the company that manufactures the prosthesis and the surgical instruments was also present—both for consultation and to monitor the operation in order to assist the nurses with the instrumentation. Dr. Wolf told me that the company representative's presence is routine because of the rapid development of new and improved instruments in joint-replacement surgery.

I was also there, trying to be as unobtrusive as possible but close enough to the action so that I could see what was going on in great detail.

Let the Surgery Begin

What follows is based on my own experience in having both knees and my left hip replaced as reconstructed from my medical records and subsequent discussions with Dr. Wolf, supplemented by the personal observation of a total knee replacement that I've just mentioned. Although no two operations are exactly the same—there are always variations depending on the condition of the patient and the particular methods of the surgeon—my experience is fairly typical of most knee- and hip-replacement patients.

Once the anesthesia has kicked in, the surgeon will position you on the operating table so that he can have the best access to the area where he'll be working. Then a large area surrounding where the incision will be is washed and covered with iodine—one of the many steps taken to guard against infection. This area is then covered with a sterile plastic sheet.

In the case of a knee replacement, a tourniquet is then wrapped around the upper thigh and the knee is flexed. The operation is now ready to begin.

The first thing the surgeon will do is open up the joint by making an incision down the middle of your leg (for a knee) or in the lower portion of your thigh (for a hip). (If you want to see exactly where and how long the scar is, just about anyone who's had a joint replacement will be happy to show you.) The skin and underlying fat and tissues are then folded back until the bones of the joint are completely exposed.

From the X rays, the surgeon usually has a pretty good idea of what he will find when the joint is open. (With my first knee replacement, Dr. Wolf's arthroscopic exam had shown

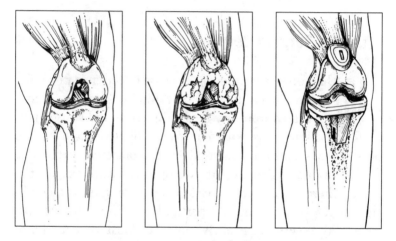

THE HEALTHY KNEE (*left*): Smooth, slippery white cartilage covers the contacting surfaces of the knee joint, permitting it to bend and straighten as much as 100 times per minute without pain.

THE ARTHRITIC KNEE (*center*): Over time, the cartilage wears away, leaving the surfaces of the joint pitted, eroded and uneven. The result is stiff, unstable movement and, of course, accompanying pain.

TOTAL KNEE REPLACEMENT (*right*): To regain smooth, pain-free movement, the end of the femur is resurfaced with a metal implant and the tibia and patella are resurfaced with plastic implants or implants made of both metal and plastic.

him that I was going to need a total knee replacement.) Still, there's nothing like seeing the condition of the joint with the naked eye. In the case of the knee-replacement surgery I was able to observe, Dr. Wolf was not certain until the patient's knee was opened up whether she would need a partial or a total knee replacement. The final decision—a total knee—was made on the operating table.

The next step is cleaning out the joint—removing torn cartilage, bone chips, and dead tissue. Then the bones that make up the joint are resurfaced. In a knee, there are three such bones: the femur (thigh bone), tibia (shin bone), and patella (kneecap). Each is approached separately and, in my case at least, in that order.

The resurfacing consists first of cutting the bone ends to remove diseased bone and shaping the bone ends so that the prosthesis will fit over them. This process, as Dr. Wolf told me the first time we talked about my having a knee replacement, is basically an exercise in "carpentry" in which the surgeon will use drills, jigs, cutting blocks, screws, saws, calipers, hammers, and other instruments. Of course, this is carpentry where you can't just start all over again if you don't get it right.

As the bone ends are cut, the surgeon will size the remaining surfaces in order to determine the size of the prosthesis that will be implanted.

Like a natural knee, the prosthesis also consists of three components.

First, there's a metal component (in my case, a titanium alloy) that is fitted onto the end of the femur. The femoral component has some studlike projections that help to fix it to the bone. Since mine is a press-fit prosthesis rather than one that is held in place by cement, the surface that is in contact with the bone is porous so the bone will grow into it.

The component which will cover the tibia is a metal plate and stem. The plate accommodates an insert made of high-density plastic—in effect, the new joint's cartilage—on which the new metal surface of the femur will rest. The stem is inserted into the tibia, where it is anchored with a press-fit process.

Finally, the kneecap is resurfaced with a circular piece of high-density plastic, which takes the place of lost cartilage and diseased bone. Unlike the other two components, the new kneecap surface is almost always cemented in place. "It's the one component," says Dr. Wolf, "that seems to do better with a cemented technique, although there are some surgeons who have had equally good results with a metal-backed, press-fit component."

Although press-fit rather than cemented prostheses are increasingly being used for both knee and hip replacements, many patients are better off with a cemented prosthesis. As a general rule, surgeons prefer to cement the prosthesis into place for patients who are older, less well, or more sedentary. Patients with medical problems might not be able to heal their bones to an ingrowth prosthesis. Loosening of a cemented prosthesis in patients with a relatively sedentary lifestyle is not likely. This is why patients with rheumatoid arthritis, whose activity levels are generally lower than those of people with osteoarthritis, are more likely to have cemented prostheses.

Another advantage of a cemented prosthesis is that the patient is able to put full weight on the replaced joint with the knowledge that the fixation is total and immediate. Biologic-ingrowth prostheses require a year for full fixation to take place. The patient can experience some level of pain until the biologic fixation is complete. Sometimes the decision of whether to cement or press-fit may be made right on the operating table. Says Dr. Wolf:

> You can tell a lot about the quality of the bone when you cut
> through it. If it's very soft and cuts very easily then the basis

on which you're going to apply a prosthesis is not good. If you have good solid bone stock to work with, it's encouraging, especially when you're using a prosthesis that needs that bone for stability without cement. If I were to find for whatever reasons during an operation—even though I may have planned to do an uncemented prosthesis—bone quality was less than I hoped, I would then cement the prosthesis.

After the prosthesis has been put into place and secured, the surgeon will wash out the entire exposed area with a saline solution—another measure to guard against infection. He's then ready to close you up. Sutures that will eventually dissolve in the body are used to sew up the various layers beneath the skin.

The final closing of the wound, however, is usually done with metal staples. I didn't even realize that I'd been stapled back together until I returned to Dr. Wolf's office to have my stitches removed and found him using a staple remover to do the job. (This sounds worse than it is.) When I asked Dr. Wolf why he used staples, he said:

Staples are extremely efficient. Sutures are much more difficult and inconsistent. Stapling a wound together is very quick. You can staple an entire wound together from one end to the other for a knee or a hip in a couple of minutes at most. Suturing would take much more time. It might take as long as five or ten minutes to suture a long wound together and it's more difficult. Staples are really what most surgeons use on large wounds that need to have separate points of closure.

In broad outline, a hip replacement follows the same general pattern as a knee replacement. The main difference is that, as mentioned earlier, a hip has only two bones: the femur, which has the ball, and the pelvis, which has the socket. A hip is also more stable than a knee since it is powered by large muscles and is secured by its ball-and-socket construction. All of this is what enables you to walk, twist, turn, and squat. Consequently, a hip replacement is actually much simpler than a knee replacement.

Once the hip joint has been completely opened, the sur-

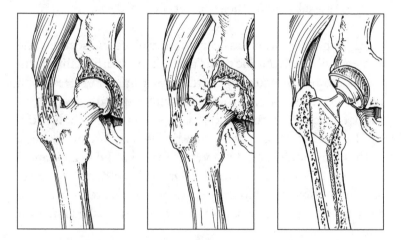

In a healthy hip (*left*), smooth cartilage covers the ends of the thighbone and pelvis. This allows the ball to glide in any direction inside the socket.

In a hip requiring total-hip-replacement surgery (*center*), the worn cartilage no longer serves as a cushion. As the damaged bones rub together, they become rough, with a surface like sandpaper. This results in pain with almost any movement, and steadily decreasing mobility.

In a total hip replacement (*right*), the ball replaces the head of the thighbone. The stem component of the ball, which is made from a superalloy material, is inserted into the thighbone for stability. A cup made out of durable white plastic material replaces the worn socket in the hip. The prosthesis is held in place either by new bone growing around it or by a cement-like material.

geon will dislocate the hip by rotating the ball out of the socket. He will then drill a hole down into the femur and ream it out, creating space for the stem of the prosthesis to rest. He will then cut off the ball at the end of the femur. Then the socket is smoothed out and shaped to hold the other part of the prosthesis.

Like a natural hip, the prosthesis also has two components. A new socket made of high-density plastic encased in metal is fitted into the pelvic indentation. This is usually secured by a press-fit process. Then the other component, a metal shaft with a metal or ceramic ball, is inserted into a hole previously drilled in the femur, and the ball and socket are joined. The ball component is sometimes secured by cement even when the socket is press-fit.

And that's it.

The typical hip or knee replacement takes about an hour and a half operating time.

(A video of a total knee replacement performed by Dr. Wolf is available through Dr. Wolf's web site: www.eugene-wolf-md.com.)

6

From Recovery Room to Discharge

T he first thing I noticed after waking up in the recovery room—and this was true for all three of my joint replacements—was that the pain was gone. I have since heard the same thing from many other joint-replacement patients.

But don't get too euphoric. Some patients wake up in considerable pain. This doesn't mean that the operation didn't work. Says Dr. Wolf:

Everybody's different. Some patients wake up and they have no pain. Others wake up and they're in terrible pain. I can't predict it. No two knees or hips are exactly the same. I tell the patients about to undergo bilateral knee replacement that the knees will be different postoperatively, even though it is the same operation performed by the same surgeon on the same patient. It's impossible to

----

predict how the knees will react. Some knees are painful and some are not.

In any event, you're not going to be completely pain-free during your recovery. What does happen in most cases, however, is that the pain you went into the operating room with will be either gone or dramatically reduced. With the surgery and the new prosthesis, that pain—caused by the loss of cartilage and the consequent friction of bone on bone—has been largely eliminated. But it will take some time before the pain resulting from the surgery will be gone.

It's better to anticipate that you're likely to wake up with some pain even though you might not feel it right away because you will still be somewhat sedated.

Of course, if you had epidural anesthesia, you will not feel anything at all in the operated area, which will still be numb. But when the anesthesia wears off and feeling returns to your limb, chances are you'll have some pain. Lady Andy had both knees replaced within a month of each other in early 1997 at the Cedars-Sinai Medical Center in Los Angeles. A week after returning home from her second knee replacement, she was back on-line again with the latest news:

This time there was more post-operative pain, but that was just one day, so not too bad. After that, the pain-medication I received by IV drip controlled it for about 3 days, then they switched me to oral pain medication (Vicodin).

Just a word of advice. After the epidural, they warned me I would need extra pain medication by injection before the drip really began to work. Boy, don't hold off on telling them you're ready for that extra injection. That was the one and only period of really bad pain. But don't be scared. After the injections and the drip began to work, there was no real bad pain again. Just don't try to be tough and wait too long to ask for it.

While you're in the recovery room, you will be under constant and close observation. Your vital signs—blood pressure, temperature, and pulse—will be regularly monitored. If you get impatient, just remember that you've been through major surgery. (Thirty years ago, after a hernia operation, I went into shock in the recovery room—possibly from the loss of blood or the trauma—and the nurses were on me quicker than you could say "Nurse!")

After a while—anywhere from one to three hours—you'll be taken to your room. The nice part about this, in addition to being on a ride less fraught than the one you took to the operating room, is that you will already be in your own bed. However comfortable you might feel, you won't relish the idea of a bed transfer at that point.

A Room of My Own—Well, Not Quite

If you're lucky, when you're wheeled into your hospital room you'll have it to yourself. Not that I'm antisocial. But the last thing you want coming out of surgery is either a chatty roommate, no matter how well intentioned, or someone with a lot of visitors who have come to cheer him up and forage through his candy. I even told my wife not to bother waiting around for me on the day of the operation since the one thing I was sure I'd want to do afterward was sleep. I'd also advise telling anyone else who might want to visit to hold off at least a day or two—unless, of course, you're the supergregarious type and you can't wait to show off your scar, or unless your idea of a good time is to bore everyone with the gory details of your ordeal.

Actually, you're going to be pretty scary-looking right after surgery. Your body will have been through a major trauma, and that's going to show up in a lack of color and drawn features in your face. Plus you'll be hooked up to so many tubes you might look like you're on life support. In addition to the IV in the back of your hand, you'll probably have a tube draining blood from your incision (a hemovac) and an oxygen tube in your nose. You might also be hooked up to a catheter—I was—since many people have difficulty urinating the first day or two after surgery. The good news is that you'll probably be a lot better than you look.

And don't count on getting anything to eat that first day— you'll probably get only some juice and maybe a small serving of Jell-O. Believe me, you won't want any more.

A small army of nurses, nurses' aides, and orderlies will be marching through your room for the first day or two. They'll be checking your blood pressure, your temperature, your pulse, and your breathing. They'll also draw some blood from a vein in your arm every day.

One of the first things I was instructed in was how to sedate myself. The process, called Patient-Controlled Analgesia (PCA), enables you to give yourself a quick dose of morphine if the pain gets too strong. All you do is press a button and the morphine flows through a tube that runs from the dispenser into your IV. For some patients this is a godsend since you don't have to ring for the nurse to get your fix. Fortunately, I rarely felt the need to push the button. And you don't have to worry about overdosing. The PCA machine has a built-in monitor which prevents that.

Much of your treatment on this and succeeding days is designed to guard against potential postop complications. So you'll get antibiotics for a couple of days (administered through your IV) in order to prevent infection in your wound and the operated area.

A lot of attention is paid to the problem of possible blood clots (embolisms) developing in your legs. During surgery, much of the blood supply to your leg is cut off by a tourniquet. And in the immediate postop period you're going to be lying in bed pretty much in one position. Those are conditions under which blood clots can form. If a large embolism breaks off and travels to your lungs, the consequences can be fatal. Blood clots are the number-one cause of postoperative death in knee and hip surgery—although such an outcome is extremely rare. Even a small clot can produce complications that can require an extended hospital stay.

Fortunately, the medical profession has developed many techniques for preventing that from happening. In addition to the surgical stockings and some initial lying-in-bed exercises, you'll probably be given some form of anticoagulant medication or a blood thinner, also through your IV. (Later, when your IV is removed, you might get this drug in the form of a small pill.)

After each of my three joint replacements, I was given a low dosage of Coumadin daily. To give you an idea of how powerful a drug it is, Coumadin is the main ingredient in the most common forms of rat poison. In small doses, it's easy to control and has proven quite effective for humans. I was on Coumadin for three or four weeks, and after I left the hospital I was monitored at home once a week by an RN from the Visiting Nurses Association of California, who would measure the effect the drug was having on my blood's clotting time.

Other postop complications can develop if your surgery was performed under general anesthesia—as all three of mine were. Under a general, parts of your lungs don't function normally during the operation and might not be functioning fully after you wake up. As a result, there is a risk of congestion or pneumonia. So you'll be given some deep breathing and coughing exercises in which you inhale deeply through your nose and exhale slowly through your mouth. You'll probably also be given a device called an incentive spirometer (sometimes called a "blow bottle") in which you elevate a little ball as high as you can with your exhaled breath. This is an exercise designed to clear your lungs and rejuvenate their functioning. You'll be urged to do this exercise several times daily for about two or three weeks.

The Continuous Passive Motion Machine (CPM)

Once I was comfortably ensconced in my bed after my first knee replacement, I noticed something peculiar. The blanket over my new knee was slowly, almost imperceptibly, moving up and down. I watched it for a while and finally called the nurse to find out what was going on.

It turns out I was hooked up to a device called a continuous passive motion (CPM) machine, which was ever so gently raising, lowering, and slightly turning my operated leg. The idea was to slowly increase my new knee's range of motion. My postop physical therapy had begun and I hadn't even known it. In addition, a cooling device was attached to the CPM and moved with it, helping to reduce the swelling in my knee.

I remained on the CPM throughout my hospital stay, and the discharge nurse arranged for me to lease the machine for my first week at home. (The cost was covered by Medicare.) The great thing about it—in addition to providing a low-level continuous exercise for my knee—is that it was so gentle and so quiet that I didn't even know it was on. In fact, when I'd wake up in the middle of the night I'd had to look at the blanket to see if it was moving in order to be certain the CPM was functioning.

Some patients, however, find it a nuisance. For one thing, you have to sleep on your back, which a lot of people can't do. This didn't bother me since I had been sleeping on my back ever since my first arthroscopic surgery. It was the only position in which I could sleep without pain. Other people complain about the noise or the motion, but I think they probably didn't get good instructions on adjusting the settings.

The one major problem in using a CPM at home is that you have to disconnect it whenever you're out of bed and then position yourself into it and reconnect it when you go back to bed. The ice supply also has to be regularly replenished. Naturally, these jobs fell to my wife, who became quite expert at it, but it was still a bit of a nuisance. After the first day at home, I decided to use the CPM only at night.

On that first day in my room, after both my knee and hip replacements, I was started on some very simple isometric exercises that I could do while lying in bed. These are so simple you might wonder how they could possibly help you, but they will. Designed to strengthen your leg and thigh muscles and reduce swelling, they're not painful (you're contracting the muscle without moving the joint), and they begin to work your muscles gently. They will also help prevent blood clots. Here they are:

Quad Sets The quads (quadriceps) are a group of muscles in the thigh that both stabilize your knee and help you move it. After surgery they need to be strengthened. Press the back of your knees down into the bed by tightening your thigh muscles. You can start by holding the position for a second or two and, as you feel up to it, increase the hold to five seconds. I did each hold five times and was told to try to repeat the exercise five times every hour.

Gluteal Sets Squeeze your buttocks together, which causes your hips to rise slightly. Again, hold the position briefly, gradually building up to a five-second hold.

The nurses suggested I do both exercises whenever I wanted, and since there wasn't much else to do anyway, I soon became a black belt in quadriceps and gluteal sets. The in-house physical therapist might prescribe some other exercises as well.

Except for the CPM machine, which was used only after my knee replacements, all these measures and exercises were part of my regimen after both my knee and hip replacements. In addition, there are certain things that are done especially for hip replacements. These are designed principally to prevent dislocation of your new hip—a serious hazard during the first six postop weeks—and especially in the first couple of

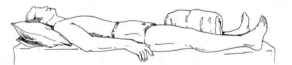

When lying on your back, keep a folded pillow between your knees.

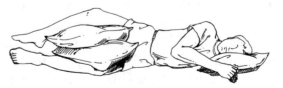

When lying on your unoperated side, place two pillows between your legs.

days—because until the prosthesis is firmly in place, it has a limited safe range of motion. Most of what I'm about to describe will take effect when you become ambulatory, but one or two things will be implemented immediately.

Thus, when I woke up from surgery after my hip replacement, I discovered that there was a triangular foam cushion wedged between my legs. This is to prevent you from crossing your legs, something we all tend to do naturally from time to time but that, with a relatively unstable new hip, can cause dislocation. Many hospitals will also put a hip-replacement patient in a bed that tilts to a standing position—usually only for the first day.

On the Comeback Trail

Aside from the simple aerobic and breathing exercises, you'll be a passive patient on that first day. Don't get too used to it. On the very next day you will move into recovery and rehabilitation mode.

To begin with, your surgeon will come to see you. By the time we got to my third joint replacement, Dr. Wolf and I had worked out a routine. He would say, "How're you doing?" and I would say, "You tell me." Fortunately, his answer was always the same: "Great!" Then I'd ask him how the surgery went and he'd get a little more detailed.

After the first operation, Dr. Wolf said putting in the new knee had been "Nothing but net!"—meaning it was a perfect fit the first time he tried it. He also told me I had really good bone structure, which enhanced the prospects for stability in my new joint and had confirmed his plan to give me a press-fit rather than a cemented prosthesis. Your surgeon will also want to know if you have any problems. Don't be bashful. This is your chance to ask any questions that have occurred to you—there are always some—and to register any complaints you might have. (Don't bother complaining about the food, though. It won't do any good!)

This is also the day you'll starting eating whole food again. Considering the usual quality of hospital food, that might not sound like much. But it's a big psychological lift, especially when the nurse gives you the menu so you can make your choices for the next day's meals. Sure, they always sound better than they turn out to be, but it's a step in regaining control over your life. And every once in a while you'll get a dish that actually tastes like it's supposed to.

Since one of the common aftereffects of surgery is some constipation for a few days, you might want to order some prune juice or prunes with your breakfast. Both are usually on the menu for that reason.

This will also be the day you'll start getting unhooked from your tubes. The oxygen feed and the catheter will probably be the first to go. The drain and the IV will likely stay in a little longer.

But for me, the really big event of the day was when the physical therapist told me I was going to get out of bed. My first reaction was "You've got to be kidding!" But he assured me he wasn't. And he wasn't. Of course, physical therapists are basically optimists; otherwise they couldn't do what they do. And you might be thinking that in your case, an undue optimism is not called for. Just keep in mind that your therapist has done this a thousand times before and probably knows more about your condition and what you're capable of than you do.

The routine of getting out of bed and taking your first steps varies from hospital to hospital and therapist to therapist, so don't be surprised if yours doesn't go exactly the same way mine did. There will also be slight variations depending on whether you've had a knee or a hip replaced.

Off the Bedpan and On to the Toilet

For most people, getting out of bed is something you just do without thinking. After a knee or hip replacement, however, even thinking about it is liable to be painful. Fortunately for those of us who have been on the replacement track, the surgeons, the nurses, and the physical therapists have given it a lot of thought. The most important thing to keep in mind is that it's a series of separate actions that have to be taken one at a time.

First you have to get into a sitting position, for which you'll probably need some assistance—especially if you've had a hip replacement. Then you've got to swing your legs around so that they're hanging over the side of the bed. (With a hip replacement, you'll probably use a special carrying device called a leg raiser so that it can be lowered gradually rather than all at once.)

At this point you'll need a little rest.

Now you're going to stand! Easier said than done, right? Not to worry. The therapist will not want you to put your full weight on the operated side and so you'll hold on to a walker or the back of a chair or even the therapist as you gradually ease down out of the bed and onto your feet. When you've done that, it will be time for another short rest and a quick round of applause from your roommate.

Next you're going to sit down. That sounds good—but how are you going to do it? Of course, the therapist has anticipated the complexity of the operation. So the chair will have arms and—especially if your hip has been replaced—will be at least twenty inches high. You'll slowly back up until your legs touch the edge of the seat and then, holding on to the arms of the chair to support your weight, you'll gradually lower yourself into it, always keeping your operated leg out in front.

By this time you'll feel as though you've done a day's work, so prepare to sit for a while. And that might be all you do until it's time to get back into bed. But for most patients, the best is still to come. You're going to walk!

In any event, you'll have to get up again. This, you'll find, is actually easier than sitting down, since you use the arms of the chair for leverage.

The main problem in walking is making sure you don't put your full weight on the side where you've had the replacement—especially if the joint has not been cemented into place. Even with cement, the leg will be pretty tender. If you're using a walker—which I would recommend except for when you have to climb and descend stairs—this is the way you'll be advised to do it: Lift the walker and place it a few inches in front of you. Leaning on the walker to support your weight, take a small step forward with your operated leg. Continuing to lean on the walker, step ahead with your "good" (unoperated) leg, bringing it parallel to or slightly ahead of the other leg. Then repeat. The same principle applies if you're using crutches.

That first step will take a while, and it will probably be painful. But once you've done it, you'll feel a great sense of accomplishment. How far you'll walk that first time out will depend mostly on the severity of the pain and how much you can bear. A good first goal is to make it to the bathroom, which will not only enable you to relieve yourself but will do wonders for your dignity. (By the next day, believe it or not, you'll probably be able to get to the bathroom on your own.)

Over the next few days you can expect to be making steady progress in being ambulatory. At first, you won't do much without the physical therapist. But pretty soon you'll venture out alone beyond the door to your room. Two days after surgery I was making friends in other rooms and comparing notes with other joint-replacement patients. By the next day I was able to make a circuit of the whole ward. One of the first rewards of being ambulatory is that you'll start taking your meals in a chair rather than in bed.

At some point I received a blood transfusion. Actually, I was getting back the blood that I had donated earlier and that was never used during surgery. There's more to this procedure than being thrifty. Since the blood carries oxygen, it will help get you pumped up and as energetic as possible.

Although I was making good progress in my walking, I was surprised when, on the day before I was scheduled to leave the hospital, the physical therapist announced that I was going to navigate stairs. We went to the physical therapy room, where I was brought to a construction consisting of four or five steps leading up to a flat area. The therapist showed me how to step away from my walker and take hold of the banister. I went up the stairs one at a time, leading with my strong (unoperated) leg. At the top I turned around and then went down, this time leading with my weak (operated) leg. It was a little intimidating at first, but after a while it got to be fun.

Joint-replacement patients using crutches actually did the same thing, learning how to tuck their crutches under one arm while they navigated the stairs. The reason patients who have stairs at home are advised to use crutches is that they can take their crutches with them when climbing or descending the stairs. That's not advisable with a walker.

At some point you'll be visited by an occupational therapist, who will instruct you in handling practical problems of everyday living such as getting dressed, putting on your shoes, tying your shoelaces, taking a shower, and so on. Concerning shoes, your best bet is to use some kind of moccasin or slip-on shoe without laces, since bringing your operated leg up to tie the shoelaces will be extremely difficult after a knee replacement and an absolute no-no after a hip replacement.

You probably won't be permitted to try taking a shower on your own. For one thing, you will have to make sure not to get the wound wet, so your operated leg will have to be wrapped in some tight-fitting, heavy-duty plastic before you're even permitted into a shower. There might also be problems getting in and out of a shower—even a stall shower—if there's any kind

Managing Stairs

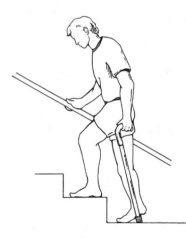

Upstairs:

a) The good (or stronger, if both knees have been replaced), leg goes first.

b) The operated (or weaker, if both knees have been replaced) leg goes second.

c) The cane goes last.

Downstairs:

a) The cane goes first.

b) The operated (or weaker, if both knees have been replaced) leg goes second.

c) The good (or stronger, if both knees have been replaced) leg goes last.

of ledge that you will have to lift your operated leg over. And then, of course, there's the danger of slipping when you're in the shower. You really shouldn't take a shower before the staples are out.

Hip-Replacement Precautions

All this is difficult enough after a knee replacement. After a hip replacement, all activity has to be thought through and anticipated in the context of special precautions to avoid dislocating your hip. This is a particular danger because, as mentioned earlier, the surgeon actually dislocates your hip during surgery. He has to do that in order to resurface the bones in the joint and to put the new prosthesis into place. Consequently, it will take some time for the components of the prosthesis to stabilize in your new hip.

This process generally takes about six weeks. During that period you will have to observe certain restrictions, the most important of which are as follows:

Don't bend your hip past a 90-degree angle. In general, aim for a 70-degree maximum bend to keep yourself well within the safety range. This means not bending down to pick up objects from the floor or from low surfaces. It also means sitting in a chair that will enable you to keep your knees level with or below your hips. Stay away from low chairs (less than eighteen inches high) or overstuffed chairs. Sinking into a couch or an overstuffed chair can immediately bring you past the danger point. And make sure whatever chair you sit in has strong arms that you can use to leverage yourself up. Otherwise you might find yourself sitting there for a long time.

Don't cross your legs—even at the ankles and especially at the knees. Sleep with the foam cushion between your legs at least until your doctor advises you it's safe not to. When you're sitting, keep both feet on the floor with your knees six to eighteen inches apart.

Don't turn the knee of your operated leg inward in a pigeon-toed position. Keep your knee pointed forward or slightly out.

Don't reach across your body. If you have to get something requiring such a motion, turn your entire body around first.

Use an elevated toilet seat or a commode that fits over the toilet. The advantage of a commode is that it has arms which you can use for help in lowering yourself and getting up. If you use an elevated toilet seat, make sure you have grab bars or some stable surface (such as a sink) next to the toilet for getting up and down. The advantage of an elevated toilet seat—that's what I used—is that it is smaller, more compact, and less expensive.

The consequences of ignoring or forgetting these precautions can be severe. Checking out my favorite arthritis news group on the Internet, I came across the following:

> The day after I got home from the hospital following my hip replacement, I really did a dumb thing. I was feeling so good that I forgot about not bending too far and I managed to dislocate my new hip completely out of the socket! Talk about pain! I made a $400 trip by ambulance to the hospital where I had the replacement done. Fortunately the doctor was able to reposition my hip without further surgery. But I was kept in the hospital overnight as a precaution.

Hip Replacement Precautions as Recommended by the Hospital for Special Surgery

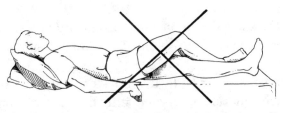

Do not cross your legs when lying, sitting, or standing.

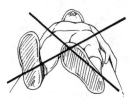

Do not roll legs inward toward each other. Your feet should be pointed up toward the ceiling or outward.

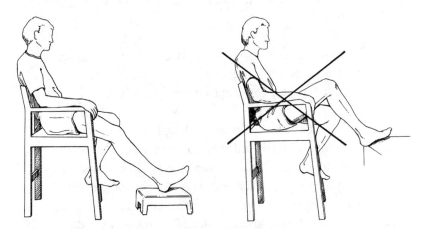

When you are sitting in a chair, the height of your knee *must* be lower than your hips. If you sit on a stool, make sure it does not raise your knee above your hip level.

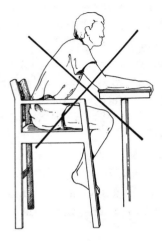

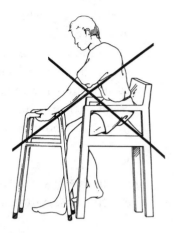

Do not lean forward past a 90-degree angle at your waist.

When rising from a chair *do not* pull up on your walker, crutches, or cane. *Do* use an armchair, so you can use the arms to push up from the chair.

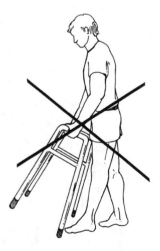

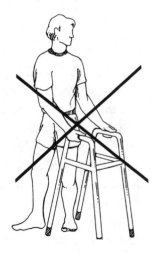

Do not take a step unless your walker is flat on the ground.

When walking with a walker, crutches, or cane, *do not* turn by pivoting on your operated leg.

The result was a small fracture in the hip that hasn't healed yet and which the doctor says may be permanent. I now have to be VERY careful, and have actually had it slide out of the socket and back in again since then. Thank goodness it has only amounted to that. Also, the muscles and tendons in that area haven't completely built back up as a result of the fracture. Still, I got off lucky and it's wonderful to be without pain in my hip.

In addition to the elevated toilet seat and the grab bars, there are a number of small appliances that will enable you to function while observing these restrictions. These include:

- A reacher, much like the device used in old-time grocery stores when the clerk had to get a can or a box down from a high shelf. Its main function is to enable you to pick up objects without bending or to grab objects that are too high. I used this one more than any of the others.

Slide the sock or stocking on to the sock aid. Make sure the heel is at the back of the plastic and the toe is tight against the end. The top of the sock should *not* come over the top of the plastic piece. Holding on to the cords, drop the sock aid out in front of the operated foot. Slip your foot into the sock aid and pull it on and then off the back of your foot.

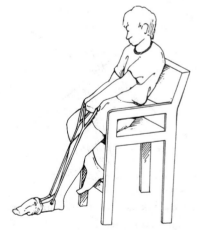

- A long-handled shoehorn for getting your foot into your shoes without going beyond the 90-degree angle.
- A sock aid. I loved this one. It enables you to put your socks on without bending over or crossing one leg over the other. You won't believe it until you try it.
- A long-handled sponge for washing your back, your feet, and other body parts without violating the hip restrictions.
- A dressing stick. This one's especially good for getting your pants on.
- A leg raiser. This one enables you to lift your leg when you're getting into bed and lower it when you're getting out.

The good news for those of us on Medicare is that Medicare paid for all of these. (I've been told that HMOs don't always cover them.) The bad news is that I didn't learn about these tools until after my hip replacement. Most of them would have stood me in good stead prior to the surgery. In fact, I could have used several before and after my knee replacements as well. Perhaps if you can get a prescription for these from a physical therapist before surgery you might be able to get some of them without charge.

If you have to buy any of this equipment, try places like Sears or JCPenney or a large, supermarket-style drugstore. (In California, Long's or Payless.) Otherwise, try a medical supply store. (These are listed under "Medical Equipment and Supplies" in the classified pages.) Keep in mind, however, that prices in the medical supply houses are usually higher. So, provided the quality is the same, you might want to get whatever you can in the larger, all-purpose stores. There are also some mail-order houses specializing in such equipment, but you'll probably do better if you can see and try the product before buying it.

For the grab bars and the more specialized items, your best bet is a place like Home Depot, where you can get the old-fashioned, strong, stainless steel kind. Medical supply houses tend to be more expensive and, I have found, do not stock the really heavy-duty kind.

The Skilled Nursing Facility

One of the first questions you will undoubtedly ask your doctor is "When can I go home?" Don't worry. The hospital doesn't want to keep you a day longer than it has to. If anything, the thing to worry about in these days of cost cutting and "customer" turnover is being sent home too soon. I hope that your surgeon won't feel unduly pressured by the hospital bureaucracy to discharge you before you're ready.

My hospital stay for each of my three joint replacements was five days—in on a Monday and out on a Friday. That was pretty much what Dr. Wolf had told me to expect going in. But I've since heard that some HMOs are trying to limit the stays of joint-replacement patients to four and even three days. It can be done, I suppose, but it will be a lot harder on you and whoever is taking care of you at home.

In fact, many joint-replacement patients don't go directly home from the hospital. Some go to a skilled nursing facility (SNF), usually an adjunct of the hospital, where they can get an additional few days of therapy. If the hospital doesn't have an SNF, you can go to a convalescent hospital. I would strongly recommend one or the other for any patient who lives alone because you will be further along in your recovery by the time you have to fend for yourself at home. But even if you've got someone else at home, it will be a lot easier on that person—particularly if, like the typical joint-replacement patient, you and your principal caregiver are in the Social Security set.

Unfortunately, I didn't learn about the availability of a skilled nursing facility until I was on my third joint replacement, which happened to be my hip. As it turns out, an SNF is generally considered more appropriate for a knee replacement than a hip replacement. Nevertheless, I went to the SNF anyway, and it was a good move.

Later on I asked Dr. Wolf why he hadn't recommended a stay at the SNF after my knee replacements. He said he thought I would do just as well at home. But he also said that in his experience many patients didn't like being in the SNF. One reason is that there are a lot of really sick people there—whereas the typical joint-replacement patient tends to be healthy.

My SNF roommate was a pretty sick guy. No one told me, but I think he had stomach or intestinal cancer. He was bedridden, in a lot of pain, and, I suspect, terminal. The curtain was usually drawn around his bed, and since he was on the window side, the room was always dark and gloomy. Not exactly an optimism-generating atmosphere.

Also, since SNF patients like myself are in the "subacute" category, I didn't get as much attention from the nurses as I had in the hospital. There were always people whose situations were more urgent than my own.

On the other hand, I got two forty-five-minute therapy sessions a day and I had the run of the ward, so I got a lot of additional exercise. There was also a pleasant TV and reading room with a small library, and I hung out there a lot. Still, I came away thinking I could have used a stay at the SNF even more after my knee replacements.

Going Home

Whether you're going home from the SNF or the hospital, discharge planning and execution are major concerns for you and the hospital staff. The two people on the hospital staff most concerned with your discharge are someone from the social service department of the hospital and the occupational therapist.

None of us wants to stay in the hospital longer than we have to. But neither should we allow ourselves to get pushed out by the financial considerations of our insurance providers or the hospital itself. And remember, even your surgeon might be under pressure to get you home early. If you don't think you're ready, you have a right to object. Or alert a family member to be prepared to object on your behalf if necessary.

Good reasons for objecting to early discharge, according to *Consumer Reports on Health*, are if you're unable to go to the bathroom unassisted, if you have problems keeping food down, if you have pain not controlled by oral medication, or if you feel faint, unsteady, or disoriented. Talk to your surgeon about this first, but if that doesn't work, discuss it with the hospital's discharge coordinator, the person from the social service department, or the patient advocate. You can also send a written appeal to your insurance carrier or the hospital administration. (It's a good idea to have someone fax this letter while you are still in the hospital.)

Once you're on record saying you don't feel ready, most hospitals are going to listen. They don't want an expensive lawsuit on their hands if you run into problems at home that might suggest they should have kept you longer.

In any event, says *Consumer Reports on Health:* "Don't leave the hospital without written instructions from your surgeon about what to do once you get home. At the very least, the instructions should list all medications you're supposed to take, including the doses and timing; any dietary restrictions; the activities you should and shouldn't do; and the schedule for follow-up visits or for resuming normal activities. Further, you should receive written instructions from the home-care department about any services you'll need from a physical therapist, visiting nurse or home health aide."

The person from the social service department will meet with you once your surgeon has set a date for your discharge. In my case, she was the person who made the arrangements with the Visiting Nurses Association of California for my home care. She will also discuss with you the mechanics of your transportation home. If someone is picking you up in a car, she will make sure the vehicle is one that you will be able to get in and out of. She'll want to know what kind of assistance you might need when you get home—especially if you have to navigate steps and whether or not the person driving you has the strength and agility to help you out of the car and to your home. If you are not being picked up, she will arrange for some other form of transportation—an ambulance or a van, for instance. She will also make sure there is someone available to get you packed up, take you through the paperwork, help you reclaim your belongings, and get you downstairs in a wheelchair.

Either the occupational therapist or the physical therapist will carefully review the process of getting you in and out of a car and will give you instruction in how to do it. When I left the hospital, the occupational therapist went down to the car with me to assist in the process.

This is especially critical after a hip replacement, since you have to observe all the appropriate restrictions while doing it. One thing is absolutely essential in this: a front (passenger) seat that tilts back and also slides back. A two-door car is generally easier to manage than a four-door car because the front seat slides back farther, giving you more room to maneuver yourself in and out. If you're tall—over six feet—and you've had a hip replacement, a two-door car might be a necessity rather than an option. Better discuss this with the hospital physical therapist and the discharge nurse beforehand. And insist on having the therapist accompany you to the car.

Warning! When you first contemplate getting into the car you're probably going to wonder why you can't just slide into the backseat (of a four-door car) and sit lengthwise, with your feet up on the seat. Don't do it! It's much too dangerous. You won't be able to wear a seat belt, and your back support will be dubious. Karen Sandy, my physical therapist, calls that a "Hail Mary!" ride and never condones it.

Also, make sure that you can get into the car from the street as opposed to the sidewalk. The sidewalk will force you to bend more. (This is even more important later, when it's time to get out.) You're going to get into the car butt first and then slowly and gingerly—you won't be able to do it any other way—scrunch yourself up on the seat until you're back far enough so that you can swing your operated leg into the car without bending it more than 90 degrees.

When I was down on the street contemplating this maneuver, my initial thought was that it was impossible. But human beings are nothing if not ingenious, and between the occupational therapist, my wife, myself, and some curious onlookers and kibitzers, the deed was done.

After that, getting out of the car on the other end was a piece of cake. The only problem was warding off the well-intentioned doorman, who most certainly would have dislocated my hip if I hadn't told him to back off.

But I was home.

CHAPTER 7

Home at Last!

There's no place like home—especially after a few days in the hospital.

But although it's great to be back in your old familiar surroundings, home can be a dangerous place for the patient recovering from joint-replacement surgery.

In chapter 4, we discussed some of the measures you could take to make your home safer after surgery. But in the preop period, those suggestions probably sound somewhat abstract because you can't fully imagine what the practical, day-to-day dangers and handicaps of functioning with a new knee or hip will be. And there is no way of knowing beforehand exactly what your physical condition will be when you get home.

But now you *are* home, and you're going to have to cope. One way to begin is to walk through a normal day's activities—room by room, action by action, step by step—as if you were doing a time-motion study. Do this, of course, with your spouse or primary caregiver and again with your physical therapist. Even if you've prepared your home beforehand, take nothing for granted. Try out everything in light of your new condition.

Be aware, however, that at this stage your main caregiver is not only your best friend but can also be your worst enemy—especially if that person is one of those people who think their role is to take care of the patient's every need.

Your safety is obviously the starting point. That should never be compromised. And you want to be as comfortable as possible. But you also want to get back on track to being self-reliant. "I'd rather do it myself" is not a knock on your caregiver. It's your declaration of independence. Besides, one of your considerations should be to ease the strains on your caregiver.

Sure, it's nice having someone at your beck and call—for a while. But it's often inconvenient, too. Your caregiver is not going to be on duty twenty-four hours a day. He or she might be on the phone or in the bathroom or out shopping just when you need something. In my case, my wife is a night person whose day rarely begins until I've already been up several hours. For example, I don't want to wait for my wife to get up before eating breakfast.

Of course, the first few days after I got home, she managed to rouse herself sufficiently to get me something to eat before flopping back into bed again. But my idea of breakfast is built around sitting at a table—I hate meals in bed—over half a grapefruit, cold cereal or a toasted English muffin, and steaming-hot black coffee while reading the *New York Times*. Besides, I hate the idea of being helpless. If you're like me—and Karen, my physical therapist, considered me a "typical" joint-replacement patient—you'll want to start functioning normally as soon as you're able—and probably a little before.

Analyzing Your Home

Let's start by taking an overall look at your home from a joint-replacement patient's perspective. To begin with, you want to be able to walk around your home safely and easily by yourself. You don't want to be forced to navigate a jumble of small objects, electrical cords, throw rugs, and other obstacles. Get rid of them—at least for the next couple of months—or tape them down.

Make sure your home is well lit. What might have been satisfactory lighting prior to your joint replacement might not be satisfactory afterward. Many homes are underlit, and the people living in them don't even know it. You might have to upgrade your ceiling lights (100-watt instead of 60- or 75-watt bulbs, for instance) to enable you to see the entire floor area clearly. Make sure the lamps are strategically placed to enhance visibility. You should especially consider lights in the closets and night-lights for when you get up to go to the bathroom or to fix yourself a middle-of-the-night snack.

Review the location of your telephones. You might want to make sure you've got a phone at your main sites—next to the bed, alongside your favorite chair, and at the kitchen table. Or get a portable phone that can fit easily into the pocket of a bathrobe. And if you don't already have call waiting or a telephone answering machine, this might be a good time to invest in one or the other—or both.

Think about what you're going to wear. Scuffs that you can easily slip into will be a lot easier than shoes with laces. And take your nonskid socks with you when you leave the hospital. I used those a lot and got an extra pair to use when the first pair was in the laundry. A bathrobe with deep pockets will be very useful for carrying objects—a book, an unopened bottle of mineral water, the mail, or that portable phone.

Pajamas can be a hassle—putting them on, taking them off, and when you use the bathroom. In fact, my main piece of clothing during the first couple of weeks—day as well as night—was a nightshirt. What you want, as the freeway signs promise, is "E-Z off and on!"

If you've got pets, proceed with care. The last thing you need is a German shepherd or even a cocker spaniel climbing all over you and trying to lick your face with an enthusiasm you could do without. And watch out for your pet cats. They always seem to think they've got the right of way and that you'll walk around them even when they're lying spread out in the middle of a narrow hallway.

Room by Room

Bedroom

The first thing you want to do is measure the height of your bed from the floor to the top of the mattress. If you've had a hip replacement, chances are your bed is too low. With the average bed, you'll probably find that your knees will go past the 90-degree threshold of safety for a replaced hip when you're sitting down.

My platform bed, which is 22 inches high, was great for me but is actually a little too high for some hip-replacement patients. The main problem with a platform bed is that during your recovery period, at least, you won't be able to make use of the drawers underneath. (Even afterward you might find that kind of bending uncomfortable.) The best bed height for a hip-replacement patient is one that lets your feet reach the floor without bringing your knees higher than your hips. Any bed less than eighteen inches high will probably be too low. If your bed is too low, you might want to have it mounted on a set of wooden blocks placed under each corner. Some people rent a hospital bed for the recovery period.

After my knee replacements I stayed on the CPM machine at night, which I think helped considerably with my recovery. But it made getting up at night to go to the bathroom too complicated. So for my first two weeks home, I used a bedpan at night.

A good-sized night table is an absolute must. You're going to want to keep a lot of stuff in easy reach: a phone, a message pad and pencil, a TV program guide and remote control, a book or a newspaper, a small pitcher of water and a glass, perhaps some medications. If the table has an easily accessible shelf, you can keep your bedpan there.

One other thing I found useful was a little dinner bell. That way, I could call for help when my wife was in another part of the house. (But don't overdo it. Remember the boy who cried "Wolf!")

Finally—and this is for hip patients—you'll need to keep your leg raiser (see page 159) within easy reach while you're in bed. Otherwise you'll find yourself stuck in bed or tempted to take undue risks trying to get in and out of bed on your own.

Room with Your Favorite Chair

This is the other room where you'll be spending the bulk of your time. So let me say right off that if you've had your hip replaced and, like me, your favorite chair is a recliner, it's probably too low. Nevertheless, the right recliner is a good chair because it enables you to keep your feet elevated. Karen Sandy explains:

Most people who undergo a hip replacement don't have chairs at home that are high enough. That usually comes as a big shock. That's why I try to get to patients at home as fast as I can because nine times out of ten I'll find them sitting in something that is really too low.

You might say, "Look, I'm not more than 90 degrees sitting in this chair." What you might not realize is that when you get up out of a chair or when you sit down, you have to lean forward, and that's where you go past the 90 degrees. And that angle becomes greater and greater the lower the chair is. If you just pile pillows up in the chair, you lose the leverage from the arms. You can't get up.

Generally, you want to have a chair that's eighteen inches in height from the floor to the surface of the seat. Then, for the average person, your hip will be higher than your knee when you're sitting. That way you'll have enough room to get in and out of the chair easily and safely. One way to solve this problem is to build up a platform made out of plywood or a simple box upside down with a lip around the edge so the chair won't slide off. Often someone in the family can make it or you can hire a carpenter to do it.

You'll also want a good-sized side table where, as with your night table, you can keep things you use all the time. Some of these may be kept in an easily reachable shelf in the table. This will help you avoid bending, stretching, and getting up and down too often. You might also want a folding tray for those times when you want to have a meal in front of the TV. And, of course, a remote control for the TV.

Finally, make sure you have a good reading lamp. One that can be adjusted easily and that has a switch within easy reach is best.

Bathroom

This is the room where you can least afford to be complacent. Almost everything you do in the bathroom is a potential

source of peril—even brushing your teeth! (Hip patients—
make sure you don't stretch across your body when you reach
for the toothpaste.)

Whether you've had a knee or a hip replacement, the first
thing you've got to do something about is the fact that your
toilet is too low. You probably discovered this even before
surgery. The answer to that problem, as already mentioned,
is either an elevated toilet seat or a commode. I had gotten a
raised toilet seat after my first knee replacement, so I stayed
with that. But Karen Sandy prefers commodes because they
have arms that will give you leverage getting up and support
sitting down. When sitting yourself down, back up against
the edge of the toilet. Then, holding on to the arms or grab
bars, slowly lower yourself onto the toilet seat, keeping your
operated leg in front of you.

Next question: Where is the toilet paper? This is one of those
questions you probably won't give any thought to until the first
time you reach for the toilet paper—and by then it's too late.
That's how I learned to pay more attention to the seemingly little details of daily life. It happened the first time I used the toilet in my new home, which I had moved into seven months
after my hip replacement. For some reason, the previous
owners had situated the toilet paper holder slightly behind the
seat on the wall to the right—which made it absolutely
impossible to get any paper without standing up and turning
my whole body around. That one got fixed in a hurry.

Grab bars are a must in the bathroom. You're probably not
going to use a raised toilet seat or commode indefinitely, but
even when you get past that stage, conveniently placed grab
bars will be a big help. Also, you're undoubtedly not going to
take a sit-down bath for at least six weeks, but you're going
to need grab bars whenever you do take a bath for the rest of
your life. You'll certainly need them if your shower is located
in the tub—and even if you have a stall shower. But don't try

to figure out where to place them by yourself. This is definitely a job for your physical therapist.

Taking a shower will always be a delicate operation—especially if you've had a hip replacement. (No shower until after the staples are removed, though.) If you have shower doors on the tub, they'll have to come off, because you won't be able to lift your operated leg high enough to step into the tub. There is a way of getting into the tub, *but don't try it on your own!*

You'll need a shower chair without arms that will be placed in the tub. (Make sure you've got a nonskid rubber mat under it.) You then back up to sit on the chair before getting into the tub. You can then bring your legs—one at a time—over the side of the tub. Your physical therapist will show you how to do this, and you should always have help doing it during your six-week period following hip-replacement surgery. The shower chair is not expensive and can be found either in a large drugstore or in such stores as Target and Wal-Mart.

You might also want to attach a hand-held shower hose and nozzle to your existing shower so that you can direct and control the flow of water while sitting on your shower seat. This is where both a long-handled brush and a long-handled sponge will come in handy. You'll also want convenient hooks for a washcloth and any long-handled implements you will use while showering.

Even a walk-in stall shower requires great caution. In most cases, you'll have to cross over a low (four-to-six-inch) ledge, which means for a split second you'll be standing on one leg in a cramped and often slippery area. That's why you'll need the grab bar. Again, get a nonskid rubber mat for the floor of the shower. Make sure you've got a ledge for soap and shampoo at the right height—and, if possible, with a lip so that the soap doesn't slide off. Even now, more than three years after my hip replacement, retrieving the soap from the shower floor after it slips out of my hand is an adventure I can do without.

Getting out of the shower is another danger point. You've got to navigate that ledge again, and this time you might not be seeing as well. If you wear glasses, you won't have them on. Maybe you got a drop of shampoo in your eye and the bathroom has steamed up. So step out carefully, using those grab bars. You'll need a bath mat, of course, *but make sure it's nonskid!* And after you've dried off and you begin to dress, move with caution. There are always some wet spots on the bathroom floor.

Kitchen

As with every other aspect of your return to functional independence, the problem of being able to use your kitchen begins with your attitude. Almost from the first day I got home after each of my joint replacements, my attitude was that the kitchen should be a normal area of activity for me. If you can manage the bathroom, I said to myself—and clearly I'd have to—there's no reason why you can't manage the kitchen. I didn't want to depend on my wife's availability in order to eat or drink; nor did I want her to feel hostage to my needs in that department.

This is another important way in which you demonstrate to yourself and to those around you that you are not an invalid. True, I couldn't and wouldn't deny the fact that there were some temporary limitations on my activity. But the challenge was to function right up to those limitations and to see how much I could push beyond them.

On the other hand, I was far from ready to resume my former role of primary household chef for dinner—the one meal my wife and I try to have together. So I wasn't thinking about any kind of extensive cooking and meal preparation. But I did want to be able to fend for myself.

If, like me, you want to be able to function on your own in your kitchen, you'll have to do some rearranging. The main thing is to make sure that everything you will need—dishes, pots, pans, foodstuffs, napkins, place mats, liquids—is easily accessible. But don't try to do this yourself! Get your spouse or a friend to move the things you're going to need most often from shelves, drawers, and cabinets that would require you either to use a ladder or to bend too far. Likewise, check out your refrigerator so that the things you will need most often are in the higher shelves.

Your reacher can help you grab small items that are too high, but—at the risk of belaboring the obvious—don't try to carry glass containers that way.

Avoid handling anything that's too big, too bulky, or too heavy. (You'll do much better with a small can of chicken broth or fruit juice than those large sizes.)

I tried to avoid cooking during the initial period of my recovery, using the microwave as much as possible for foods that required cooking or heating. But keep it simple.

Get a couple of aprons with deep pockets so that you can keep your hands free to hold on to your walker, crutches, or cane as you move around. (You'll want more than one so you can still have one while the other is in the laundry.) Karen Sandy recommends a rolling tea cart for carrying things, with the cart replacing your walker. (I attached a small basket to my walker, but Karen warns that people who do that have a tendency to overload the basket, which can cause the walker to tip over—something, I have to report, I discovered for myself.)

Another useful device is a long-handled dustpan. Sooner or later, you *are* going to drop something breakable, and you should be able to pick it up and get it out of your way at once.

Finally, for you hip-replacement patients, make sure that you've got a kitchen chair that's high enough for you to sit comfortably at the table without going past your 90-degree-bend restriction. (A couple of firm pillows might do the job here.)

Stairs

Make sure your stairs—outside the house as well as inside—are safe. A banister is essential. *Do not try to navigate stairs without one!* You must have something strong and stable to hold on to while you're going up or down stairs. If you have a staircase without a banister, either install one or do not use those stairs. And don't overlook outside steps leading up (or down) to your house. Whether you have to navigate two steps or twenty, you must have a railing to hold on to.

Everyone who lives in your home must understand the importance of not leaving objects—no matter how small or large—on the stairs. The stairs should not become an obstacle course where you have to maneuver around a book, an odd piece of clothing, an eyeglass case, mail, and a dustpan. Everyone should remember that it won't be a simple matter for you to get any of those objects out of your path and it will be extremely dangerous if you have to let go of the banister in order to walk around them. Small objects—a pencil, for instance—can likewise be extremely dangerous. If you inadvertently step on something like that you can lose your balance and go tumbling down the stairs, breaking a bone or dislocating your hip.

In chapter 4, we noted why your choice of whether to use a walker or crutches after joint-replacement surgery depends, to a great extent, on whether or not you're going to have to deal with stairs. You can't use a walker on stairs but you can use crutches. (How that's done is discussed in chapter 6, but your therapist will give you detailed instructions and will walk you through the process several times.)

On the other hand, you probably will be able to navigate stairs—at least after a week or two—just by using the banister for support and balance. The problem with a walker, though, is how you get it to the next floor. You can fold it up and tuck it under your other arm, but even folded walkers are more cumbersome to carry this way than crutches. So, if you're only using a walker and you do have stairs, someone might have to bring your walker to you when you get where you're going, or you could have one for each floor.

Do the stairs one step at a time rather than one leg after the other. Going up stairs, for instance, you would put your unoperated leg on the next step first, using the banister to keep your balance. Then, with your weight shifted to the unoperated leg, you bring up your operated leg to join the good one. Going down stairs, you reverse the process, starting down with the operated leg.

Home Alone

If you live alone, the immediate postop period will be more difficult, but doable. The first thing I would advise is to go to a skilled nursing facility (SNF) after you're discharged from the hospital. Discuss this with your surgeon and your insurer even before surgery. If you're on Medicare, your surgeon's recommendation should be enough for your stay there to be covered. On the other hand, I've heard stories about some HMOs whose policy is to approve an SNF only for people who are completely nonambulatory.

The chief value of an SNF, in addition to the more intensive program of therapy there than you would get at home, is that you will be much further along in your rehabilitation and therefore better able to function on your own by the time you get home. If you can't get into an SNF, you might look into a convalescent hospital, where, at least, you won't have to worry about cooking, cleaning, and the chores of daily living at home. Your HMO might not pay for it, but you could still get "at home" nurse assistance, which your insurance should cover.

In addition, arrange beforehand for whatever help you can get. See if you can get a relative or close friend to stay with you, at least for the first week—especially if you're not able to get into an SNF. (Even if that person works and can only stay with you overnight from dinnertime to breakfast, this will be a big plus.) If different friends are in a position to prepare meals, do shopping or laundry, help you get dressed—don't be a martyr. Accept graciously, keeping in mind, of course, that there are always going to be some "helpers" who are going to be more trouble than they're worth.

Finally, stock up beforehand on daily necessities—bottled water, toilet paper, tissues, canned goods, and prepared heat-and-serve meals. Look into Meals-on-Wheels or other meal services which will deliver a full meal to your home. The social services or senior citizens agencies of your city or county government will give you information on these as well as other services available to you.

Visiting Nurses

After each of my joint replacements, I had regular visits at home by a physical therapist, a registered nurse, and a home health aide, all supplied by the Visiting Nurses Association (VNA) of Northern California. This service was covered by Medicare. Most HMOs will also provide these services for their hip- and knee-replacement patients.

The first person to see me when I came home after my first knee replacement was Karen Sandy, my physical therapist. I fell in love with her immediately. A no-nonsense, take-charge person, Karen inspired confidence from the beginning. You knew right away that she had thought a lot about her work and that she picked up on everything. She clearly knew her stuff. But she didn't go by the book; she went by the patient.

Making sure that my wife was in on the discussion, Karen explained that this first visit was to enable her to make an over-all evaluation of my condition and my physical surroundings and that she would be designing a regimen of rehabilitation based on what she observed. The VNA plan, she said, was for her to see me three days a week for the next four weeks. If at all possible, make sure your spouse or primary caregiver is in on this initial discussion. They need to know everything you need to know about your condition, your medications, and your surroundings.

Karen then examined my knee, testing its flexion (80 degrees that first time) and range of motion. Then she had me go through all the various motions I did during the day: walking (I was using a walker), sitting, standing up, getting in and out of bed, and so on, offering comments as we went and pre-scribing an initial program of isometric exercises.

Two years later, when I started writing this book, I asked Karen about the range of conditions she encountered when she first visited joint-replacement patients. Her answer is something every one of us facing a knee or hip replacement should find useful:

> Those in the best condition were usually in fairly good physical condition prior to the surgery. Maybe their arthritis has come on more quickly and knowing they're going to need it eventually they've made an earlier decision to have a replacement. People in that range generally do better because their knee usually isn't as weak. This is what I'm guessing because I don't get to see them that much pre-operatively. People who've had a replacement because of osteoarthritis are usually happy after the surgery because the pain is a different kind of pain and they feel so much better. The people who have waited a very long time— maybe they are ill or afraid, maybe they had other things that had to be done first, maybe they had no one in the family who could help them at the time—tend to have a more difficult recovery because generally the whole body is in a weaker state. They haven't been able to be as active and the muscles around the affected joint are weaker.
>
> The people who have the most problems are usually the very elderly. Physically they tend to be more deconditioned and they may be somewhat out of it mentally. They may have a difficult time remembering directions—especially the hip precautions. Some of the younger patients don't listen or just don't care and dislocate their hips because they didn't follow the directions.

Before leaving, Karen walked us through every room of my house, identifying the danger spots and making suggestions for how to manage them. (Karen's approach to in-home physical therapy—both practical and psychological—and my experiences with it are the focus of the next chapter.)

The RN came once a week. Her function was to monitor my vital signs—blood pressure, pulse, and temperature—check the wound, and take a tiny blood sample. The main purpose of the blood sample was to measure the time it took my blood to clot (protime). This was done because I was still taking an anti-coagulant (Coumadin) to guard against embolisms in my leg. If the time went below or above certain parameters, the nurse would immediately report this to my surgeon, who might alter the dosage or switch to some other kind of medication. Fortunately, my blood always registered within the acceptable range.

The RN might also be the person who removes the staples from your incision—usually about ten days after surgery. (Dr. Wolf removed the staples after my knee replacements; the RN removed them after my hip replacement. I think Dr. Wolf did the knees because he also wanted to look at them himself since knee replacement is the more complex of the operations.) Karen tells me that the physical therapists at VNA now also do staple removals.

Home Health Aide

The VNA also supplied a home health aide, who came to see me three times a week for about four weeks. Her job is to provide patients with personal care they cannot do themselves. According to a VNA guideline given to all patients, here's what the Home Health Aide may and may not do:

The Home Health Aide *may:*
- assist with personal care such as bathing, shampooing, grooming and dressing
- assist with transfers, prescribed exercises, and walking
- do skin care and apply lotion
- assist with self-administered medications
- change bed linens
- assist with use of bedpan, bedside commode, or bathroom
- shave with electric razor
- assist with range-of-motion exercises under the direction of a nurse or therapist
- take and record vital signs
- do meal preparation, feeding, and light grocery shopping
- assist with light housekeeping
- perform additional services as instructed by the nurse or therapist

The Home Health Aide *may not:*
- give or apply medications of any kind or perform treatments such as enemas
- perform heavy housekeeping or janitorial work such as floor-scrubbing and waxing on hands and knees, washing walls or windows, cleaning ovens and refrigerator, moving heavy objects, doing heavy laundry loads, performing any activity necessitating standing on a chair or ladder
- clip toenails, trim corns or calluses, cut hair
- purchase alcoholic beverages
- handle finances such as banking, cashing checks, or paying bills or rent
- accompany patients to the doctor, dentist, etc.
- drive the patient's car or transport the patient in the aide's car

- lift heavy bedridden patients alone
- wash dishes or clean for the entire household or guests
- make personal telephone calls
- watch TV or smoke in a patient's home
- give out her home phone number or visit any other hours than regularly scheduled
- accept gifts from patients

After all three surgeries, the main thing I needed my home health aide for was to help me with bathing. Elena is a recent immigrant from the former Soviet Union, and she approached her job with typical Russian zeal. Not that she wasn't careful in helping me get in and out of the tub—the hardest part of the whole operation. Elena was big and strong, so the only risks were to my modesty, but it's amazing how easily that recedes when you're being helped to recover from surgery, especially since Elena herself had no compunctions about washing every crease and crevice of my body.

I didn't have a bath, of course. Even with Elena's help, there was no way during those first weeks after both my knee and hip replacements that I was going to risk that. But I had a shower bench and a shower hose (as described above), and once I was sure all of us were comfortable with the arrangement, looked forward to my three weekly sessions in the tub with Elena.

By the end of four weeks I could manage the whole shower operation on my own. Fortunately, my new house has a stall shower. But I do miss taking a sit-down bath—especially when I'm feeling stiff and achy after a long walk. And every once in a while I take the plunge, so to speak. But getting out of a tub—even with grab bars—is still very awkward for me, so I almost always take a shower.

Seeing the Doctor

Your surgeon will most probably want to see you ten days to two weeks after your joint replacement. If it hasn't already been done by your visiting RN, that's when your staples will be removed. But the main thing the doctor will be looking for is your general postop condition. He'll check the wound to see if there's any sign of infection—"That's our main concern in the postoperative period," says Dr. Wolf—and also look for undue swelling. There he's concerned about blood clots forming in the leg.

You'll have to be transported to your first postop doctor visit, most likely by your spouse or a friend. (You won't be ready to drive that soon.) If you can't arrange for a ride on your own, your insurance will most likely cover the cost of an ambulance or a car service. This will give you a chance to try out your new skills at getting in and out of cars. Remember, especially if you've had a hip replaced, make use of a two-door car if you can.

Your best bet is to sit in the passenger seat with a pillow or two under you. The seat itself should be pushed back as far as possible to give you maximum legroom. Also, get the seat into a semireclining position.

You should have your handicapped parking placard by this time so that your driver can park close to the doctor's office and leave the car either in a designated handicapped parking space or at a meter. That way he or she can accompany you to and from the doctor's office.

When you get to your destination, be sure to tell the driver not to park too close to the curb. You want to be able to step down to the street level rather than the sidewalk level. At sidewalk level your knees will be too scrunched up—past the danger point for hip replacements and, at the least, extremely awkward and uncomfortable for knee replacements.

What's your surgeon looking for during that first postop visit? Here's what Dr. Wolf wrote in my medical record on my first visit after my left knee replacement.

> Irwin is two weeks status post left total knee arthroplasty. He is on Coumadin, 5 mg. a day. His prothrombin yesterday was 18, normal is 12.3. [This is at the high end of the scale, indicating a longer than average time for the blood to clot. But Dr. Wolf apparently felt it was acceptable because he didn't change the prescription—IS] He is ambulating well with the walker. He is working on passive range of motion exercises at home and with a formal therapist. On exam he lacks about five degrees of full extension. He has good quadriceps control and flexes to 90 degrees. His wounds are well-healed. Staples are removed. He is doing very well at this time. He will be seen again in two weeks. X-rays today show good position of the component [the artificial knee].

Six weeks later Dr. Wolf noted that my knee was flexing to 120 degrees but that I was already reporting significant pain from my hip. It was at that time that my left hip replacement was scheduled for March 7, 1994.

I don't know how typical Dr. Wolf's postop schedule of visits is. After my hip replacement, when my staples were removed by the RN at my home, I saw him after two weeks, six weeks, three months, and nine months. Of course, I could schedule an appointment when I thought there was a problem. The only time that happened, though, was about two and a half years later, when I thought my other hip might be sending me signals that a replacement was on the immediate agenda. Fortunately, another set of X rays showed that my condition was basically unchanged since the last X rays were taken and that my fears were a false alarm. But while he had me in X ray, Dr. Wolf also got pictures of my existing prostheses, all of which, he told me, were doing well.

One Leg Longer?

One of the postop consequences of a hip replacement is that the leg on the operated side might get longer. That's what happened to me, but I didn't really notice a problem until after I switched from a walker to a cane. According to Dr. Wolf, "the hip is almost invariably made longer with a hip replacement." In most cases, he said, the difference is less than half an inch and the patient doesn't even notice it. But I noticed it—actually, my wife did, asking why I was walking so funny—and when Dr. Wolf measured it he found that my left leg had become three-quarters of an inch longer than my right.

Strangely enough, many people who have not been warned about this possibility think that, for some reason, their unoperated leg has gotten shorter. That could happen, of course, but not from the hip replacement. Remember, your new hip has replaced a worn-out and weakened joint that has lost its cartilage. The prosthesis itself probably accounts for most of the change; plus, weakened muscles have been strengthened.

Left untreated, the disparity can lead to back pain as well as abnormal wear on all your other joints. Fortunately, there's a simple solution: shoe lifts. Dr. Wolf suggested I get all my right shoes lifted five eighths of an inch. (Apparently, he likes to make the correction slightly less than the actual discrepancy.) Any good shoemaker can install lifts. Prices might vary from one shoemaker to another, but expect to spend in the neighborhood of $25 to $30 per shoe. You have to get lifts put in all your shoes—*and sneakers*—so it can begin to add up.

This will encourage you to cut back on the pairs of shoes you maintain in your wardrobe. I've got it pretty much down to a pair of dress blacks, a pair of browns, and my tennis sneakers.

The other piece of "good news" is that when you have your other hip replaced—Dr. Wolf says that for 90 percent of those who have a hip replacement, the word is *when*, not *if*—it will probably all even out.

When Can I Drive?

That's probably one of the first and most frequently asked questions every knee- and hip-replacement patient has. It's a question, Karen Sandy told me, she likes to have her patients ask because it's an indicator of their attitude. Someone who wants to know how soon he or she can drive is expressing a desire to get out of the passive mode and begin functioning independently again.

The answer is simple: When it's safe.

There are many variables in determining when it will be safe for you to drive. If you've had a hip replacement, most therapists won't want you driving until at least six weeks after surgery. A replacement knee can usually function in a car sooner, but much depends on whether it's your left or right knee. If you've had your left knee replaced, you obviously can manage sooner. I've heard of people with left-knee replacements driving three weeks postop. (That's driving an automatic; a stick shift would take longer.) It took me about six weeks after my right knee was replaced and four after my left knee.

Don't decide this on your own! Get a clearance from either your therapist or your doctor.

The Road to Recovery

Y ou're home. Your stitches are out. The pain has begun to recede. There are no significant complications from your surgery. You're moving around your house. Your physical therapist has started you on a regimen of exercises.

You are now at a crucial point in the whole joint-replacement process. In the period leading up to your surgery, the main focus of your life was on your pain, your lack of mobility, and all the things you could no longer do. Then your focus shifted to the surgery, the hospital, and your immediate postop recovery.

Now the main focus of your life will be on your physical rehabilitation. Your surgeon has done what he can. Your physical therapist can get you started and show you what to do. But how fast you recover, how well you recover, and especially the extent to which you are able to resume a normal life are principally up to you.

It all begins with attitude. I am, by nature, an optimistic person. But over time, with my ability to function compromised by pain and a sense of helplessness in the face of it, I found myself increasingly falling into a pessimistic attitude about myself, about life, and about the world in general. As my activity became more and more restricted, daily life became a frustrating and losing struggle to hold on to the shreds of my rapidly fading sense of self-sufficiency and dignity.

For any of us in this situation, the decision to go ahead with joint replacement is an important step, not only physically but psychologically. By refusing to give in to the fears of surgery and agreeing to run its risks, we have proclaimed that we are not resigned to the hand that fate has dealt us.

That decision is a declaration of optimism. But it's only the first step on the road back. Major surgery—and that's what you've just gone through—inevitably puts you in a passive role. You're on the operating table. You're under anesthesia. You're not doing, you're being done to. And even though you began to take some limited responsibility for your recovery while you were in the hospital, you were still in passive mode.

And passivity has its attractions. Invalids get attention. They get sympathy. People bring them things. They're allowed to indulge themselves. They're always being asked how they feel. Friends ask how they can help. And it's nice to be waited on—at least for a while.

The danger in all this is that you will slip into a passive approach to your rehabilitation. Karen, my physical therapist, says:

A lot of patients have been disabled for so long, they can't imagine having a normal life again. Often when I talk to them about the possibilities and goals, they'll say: "You mean I'll be able to do more than get around the house okay?" They've been in so much pain that they're happy with just a small goal.

There was a time, perhaps, when just being able to function again at a minimal level would have been considered a great accomplishment. Today there is no reason to settle for such a limited goal. That's all too easy to do, however. For rehabilitation, if it is to be successful, is hard work, and you're probably feeling somewhat sorry for yourself anyway. So it wouldn't be surprising if you gave in to the temptation to be satisfied with halfhearted efforts.

Don't do it. That's a victim's mentality. You are the responsible person now, the one who will be in charge of getting yourself well. Remember, you're not sick. Your decision to undergo surgery was an aggressive act of affirmation. Now you're going to need that aggressive attitude more than ever. For whether it's following an exercise regimen or pushing yourself to activity— walking, shopping, preparing a meal, doing the laundry or the dishes, dressing yourself—rehabilitation is a day-in, day-out process in which you constantly force yourself to take as much personal responsibility for your life as you possibly can and in which you are always looking to expand those possibilities.

Goals

When Karen Sandy first came to see me at my home, she asked me what my goals were. After a few moments, I declared with a show of optimism that was part bravado and part wishful thinking, "Playing tennis again." Karen thought about that for a moment, smiled, and simply said, "That's possible!" (I think that's when I fell in love.)

Actually, my most important and motivating goal—as it would be for most people—was being able to get back to work. Although I'm a writer, which mostly means sitting in front of my computer, my preop condition had placed me in the position where even that had become increasingly difficult. First of all, sitting in one place for stretches of time even as short as fifteen minutes had become extremely uncomfortable. Plus, my kind of writing involves research, which can't always be done sitting down. It means getting up to go to the bookshelves or a filing cabinet or to plow through old magazines when the last thing in the world you want to do is get up out of your chair. Then, of course, there's traveling to libraries and interviews.

But I never thought of getting back to work as a goal so much as a given. That's who I am and what I do.

On the other hand, tennis has always been one of my rewards for working. Now it was also my way of saying that I wanted to get back to a physical condition that would make me able not just to play tennis again but to enjoy the quality of life and independence I used to have. That, of course, was my real goal. Tennis would be icing on the cake.

Later on, when I discussed this question of goals with Karen, she said:

> Most people with joint replacements want to return to at least being independent in their daily life. Whether or not they return to sports is an individual thing. After all, you're not going to make someone into an athlete who hasn't been one before. But people need goals in order to be motivated. That's one of the biggest things. If someone has no goal, I usually have a very hard time being effective and helping them get well. But when they tell me what their goals are, I can tell them, "Okay, but this is what it's gonna take." So they know up front what they have to do to achieve that goal. That makes it concrete and they can see it's possible.

The biggest problem with long-term goals, however, is obvious—they take too long! You need them to remind you where you're going and to keep you on track. But you also need short-term goals, tangible objectives that you can reach over the short haul. After all, if you're not even able to get out of bed by yourself when you get home from the hospital, it's hard to keep focused on playing tennis again. At that point you might be thinking that you're never going to do much of anything, let alone play tennis. So you need short-term goals—like being able to get out of bed by yourself.

During the first six weeks postop, I built my life around short-term goals and used them as landmarks of progress: putting on my pants myself; taking a shower by myself; reaching 100 degrees of flexion (the degree to which you can bend your joint) on my knee; trading in my walker for a cane; getting back on my exercise bike; and, of course, driving.

Reaching one of these goals became a cause for celebration that I shared with my wife and whoever happened to be visiting at the time. The first time I could tie my own shoelaces I opened a special bottle of wine I'd been saving as I announced my new accomplishment at dinner that night. Putting on my pants *while standing up* was a big one, commemorated with a snifter of Courvoisier. It didn't take long for the others around me to get into the spirit—and spirits—of the occasions. (Of course, if you're still taking medications that require you to avoid alcohol, you'll have to settle for mineral water or juice while everyone else drinks the harder stuff.)

There's no mystery about the common thread in all this: self-sufficiency. Every little thing you can do now that you had difficulty doing before is progress toward this goal. It is something you have achieved—the payoff for the effort and discipline you are putting into your rehabilitation.

I was reasonably self-sufficient about six months after the

last of my three joint replacements. But it was a year before I could venture back onto the tennis courts—and another year before I felt that my partners had stopped feeling sorry for me.

However, I was coming back from a year of an almost continuous pattern of surgery-therapy-rehabilitation, followed by preparation for the next round of surgery. On the other hand, I was one of those highly motivated people who walk the extra mile whenever possible.

Physical Therapy

During the first four or five postop months, your program of physical therapy will be the centerpiece of your rehabilitation. You'll be instructed in specific exercises designed to restore strength and mobility to the muscles and ligaments surrounding your new joint and to get your body used to the prosthesis.

This is a lengthy process, and although you want to be careful not to go too fast, the main danger you actually face is that of unrealistic expectations. If you start out thinking you're going to be as good as new in a month or so, you can easily get discouraged. This is why short-term goals are so important. They help you realize and measure the progress you're making.

For the same reasons, avoid making comparisons between your rate of progress and that of others. Every patient and every surgery are different; measuring your progress against others' might cause you unwarranted anxiety.

Many people in the first flush of commitment after getting a new joint start off doing their exercises faithfully. But after a while there may be a letdown. One of the early-warning signs of backsliding is when you start doing your exercises only when the therapist is there. From there it's just one small step to discontinuing your exercises after the therapist no longer visits. Chances are you'll still "recover"—that is, you'll be functional once again. But it will probably take longer and not be as thorough a recovery. And you'll be less likely to make regular exercise a basic component of your life afterward.

Physical therapy after a joint replacement is a process that actually begins before your surgery and continues for a considerable time beyond. That process can be broken down into six broad stages: preop; in the hospital; in the skilled nursing facility (SNF); at home; as an outpatient; on your own. We've already gone over the first three in previous chapters:

Preop Special exercises prior to surgery, which a physical therapist can prescribe that will strengthen your muscles and bone structure and therefore speed your recovery. (See chapter 4.)

In the Hospital Most knee-replacement patients begin their in-hospital therapy with the continuous passive motion machine (CPM). Therapy under the supervision of a physical therapist starts for both knee- and hip-replacement patients the day after surgery. The main goal is to get you ambulatory so you can go home. (See chapter 6.)

In the Skilled Nursing Facility (SNF) This is additional therapy—and rest—for patients who are not quite ready to go home and who need supervised therapy every day in an SNF or the sub-acute-care section of the hospital. It's often especially helpful for people who live alone, and is usually more beneficial for people with knee replacements than those with hip replacements. If you're on Medicare, your doctor's prescription is usually enough. HMOs tend to limit use of SNFs to patients who are not ambulatory. (See chapter 6.)

In this chapter we want to focus on the therapy you will do at home under the supervision of a visiting physical therapist.

Therapy at Home

I f you're in an HMO, it will either provide or pay for this service. Dr. Wolf directs his Medicare patients to the Visiting Nurses Association (VNA) of California, which assigned Karen Sandy as my therapist. Karen came to see me at home three times a week for four weeks.

You might not be able to get that much attention these days. Karen says:

> It's no longer up to me and the doctor how much therapy you have. Now most HMOs have a ballpark figure of six home visits. So even if the doctor and the therapist agree that you need additional at-home therapy, we have to justify it and get the company's approval. Medicare will cover home visits by a therapist so long as you are homebound, which is defined to mean that it would require such a taxing effort on your part to travel to an outpatient physical therapy facility that you couldn't tolerate the exercise program.

After you get home, and for the next four weeks or so, your physical therapist will be your best friend. She will design and monitor an exercise program based not on a general set of rules but on your specific, individual condition. She will make sure you're using your walker or crutches properly, check out your furniture and your toilet arrangements, teach you how to walk and how to manage both in your house and out on the street, and, in general, measure your progress. Or, as Karen puts it:

> Your physical therapist has to be a motivator, someone who encourages you by telling you when things are going well

and knows when to call the doctor if need be. She has to be able to anticipate problems and help you avoid them. She has to reassure you when think you can't go on and when you are having too much pain. She will be your main resource for information during this period. Over and above the exercises, the physical therapist's role is to return you to the maximal possible level of independent living and functioning.

For all that, the success of your physical therapy is still fundamentally up to you. As I said before, it's all a matter of attitude. If you're one of those people who exercise only when the therapist comes, your recovery will be slower and maybe not as complete.

The exercises that follow are intended to supplement your in-home physical therapy program, especially if you want and can handle more activity. But go over them with your physical therapist before trying them. If, for some reason, you don't have a program of physical therapy at home, discuss them with your doctor or the physical therapist at the hospital.

Exercises

Ideally, you should do your entire program of exercises at least three times a day, allowing thirty to forty-five minutes per session. I did that on my more ambitious days. Mostly I did them twice a day. But don't let a day go by without doing your exercises at all.

Over the years, physical therapists have developed many simple exercises for knee- and hip-replacement patients. Some of them are equally useful for the knee and the hip. Some are particular to each joint.

To begin with, go back to the two isometric exercises (pages 146–47) in chapter 6: the quad sets and the gluteal sets. These are always good to start with.

Here are a few more simple ones:

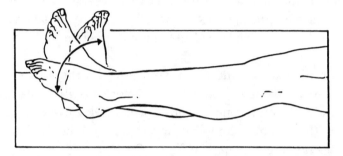

Ankle Pumps (for the hip and knee) Using your ankles to flex your feet, point your feet toward you and away from you.

Hamstring Sets (for the hip and knee) Lying flat on your back, slightly bend your knees and push your heels down into the bed as if to bend your knees. This exercise will tighten the muscles on the backs of your thighs.

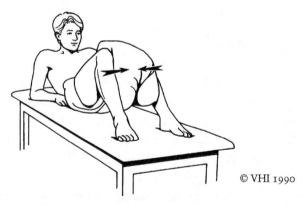

© VHI 1990

Isometric Hip Abduction (for hip and knee) Lie on your back with your knees bent. Place a folded pillow between your knees and squeeze your knees together.

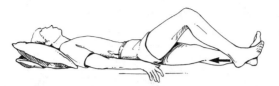

Simple Knee Bend (for hip and knee) Lying on your back, bend the knee and hip on your operated side to about 40 to 45 degrees. Hold for six seconds. Slowly lower your leg and relax.

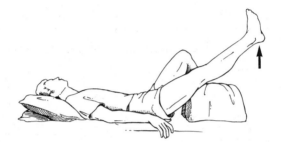

Straight Leg Raise (for hip) Lying on your back, place a pillow between your legs. Bend the unoperated leg with foot flat on bed. Raise the operated leg, keeping it straight, to height of pillow. Hold for one second and slowly lower, keeping the leg straight. (If you experience any groin pain, discontinue and try again three to seven days later.)

You'll also be given some exercises to restore flexion and range of motion. Your initial goal in flexion (how far you can bend your knee) will probably be to get back to 90 degrees. Ultimately, you should be able to get to 120 degrees and beyond. Range of motion refers to all the movements that a joint is capable of performing. You may not be able to get back to what you were able to do in the past, but you certainly should be able to improve considerably over where you were just before surgery.

Here are some more exercises you might want to try, but check with your physical therapist first.

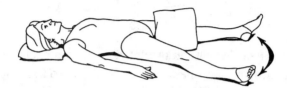

Hip Abduction (for hip) Lie on your back with a pillow between your legs. Keeping both legs straight, slide your operated leg out to the side, keeping your toes and kneecaps pointed directly up toward the ceiling. Hold for one second and return. (Ten times.)

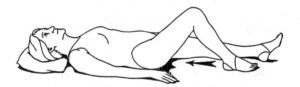

Heel Slide (knee flexion, for knee or hip) Slide the heel of the operated leg up toward your buttocks, keeping your heel on the bed and keeping the other leg flat; then slide back. If you've had a hip replacement, make sure you don't bend your hip past 45 degrees.

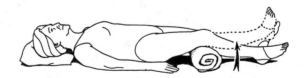

Short Arc Quads (for knee or hip) Roll up a towel or bunch up two pillows and place under the back of your operated leg;

straighten the leg and hold for two seconds; lower slowly. (Ten times.) After a while, you can build up the time of the hold.

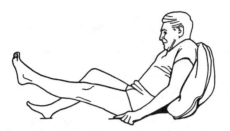

Straight Leg Raise (for knee) Lying against a pillow, bend the unoperated leg. Keep the operated leg as straight as possible and tighten the muscles on top of the thigh. Slowly lift the operated leg eight to ten inches and hold for two seconds. Slowly lower the leg to the bed, keep it tight for two more seconds, and relax.

After you've been home a few days, you're going to be spending more and more of your time out of bed—sitting, standing, and walking. As you get increasingly stable on your feet, your therapist will start giving you sitting and standing exercises. Most of these are applicable for both knee and hip replacements, always keeping in mind the hip precautions: Don't bend your hip past a 90-degree angle; don't cross your legs even at the ankles and especially at the knees; don't turn the knee of your operated leg inward in a pigeon-toed position; don't reach across your body.

These are the exercises I did: Do them standing at a counter or table, ten times each, three times a day.

Hip Abduction (standing) Stand, holding on to a counter or table for support and balance. Bring your operated leg out to the

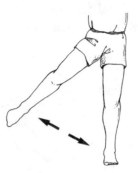

side without letting it come forward. Hold for five seconds, then slowly relax.

Following are variations on the above:

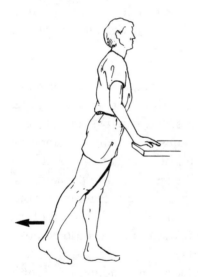

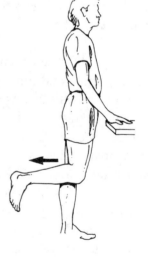

Lift your leg behind you without bending your knee; hold for two seconds, and release.

Bend your knee behind you as though you were trying to kick yourself in the butt with your heel.

Heel Lifts Lift your heel while keeping the front of your foot on the floor.

Partial Squats Bend your knees slightly, lowering your butt four to six inches.

Sitting Exercises

Sitting Knee Extension (for knees and hips) Sitting in a high chair, slowly straighten your operated leg, then lower. Hold for a count of six, then slowly lower leg so that knee is bent.

Seated back in the chair so that your thigh is supported, bend your knee as far as you can until your foot rests lightly on the floor. Then slide your upper body forward to increase the knee bend.

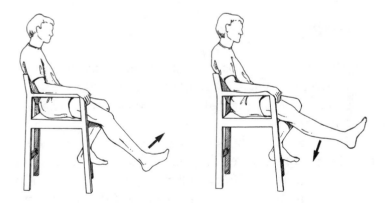

Later on, your therapist might prescribe resistance exercises by adding ankle weights, starting with a pound and perhaps working up to six or seven pounds.

One of the biggest obstacles to sticking to your exercise program is pain. This is especially true after a knee replacement, more so than with a hip. Usually you're told to discontinue any exercise when the pain gets too strong. But therapists consider these exercises so important they will often suggest you take a pain pill a half hour to forty-five minutes before beginning your exercises. (In keeping with my feeling on adopting an aggressive attitude, I prefer to call them "antipain pills.") I found that two tablets of nonprescription aspirin, Tylenol, or ibuprofen was sufficient. (*Note:* if you are taking Coumadin or any other blood thinner, don't take aspirin. If you are taking other medication, check with your doctor or pharmacist.) This won't completely eradicate your pain, but it should take the edge off enough so that you can bend your knees in the exercises even more than you would otherwise. It's also a good idea to put an ice pack on your knees for twenty minutes when you're done.

Walking

There's a lot more to rehabilitation than simply doing your exercises, though. Getting back to an active lifestyle is not only a goal, it is also part of the physical rehabilitation process.

Walking is one of the best things you can do. It's excellent exercise for a new knee or hip and the key to regaining control over your life. Almost as soon as I got home, I found any excuse I could to walk. For instance, after the first few days I started to make my own breakfast. In part this was because I didn't want to have to wait for my wife to do it. But I also derived great satisfaction from the activity itself.

I'd have to move around the kitchen to get things out of

the refrigerator, get cups and plates from their shelves, bring the toast and jam to the table—and all the other little things you do in the course of a normal activity such as preparing a meal. At first, it was somewhat frustrating being able to bring only one or two things to the dining room table at a time. But then I realized that an extra trip was an extra round of walking exercise, so sometimes I would deliberately take less than I could handle just to increase my walking time.

If someone knocked at the door, I went to answer it. I'd bring the newspaper in each morning, using my reacher to pick it up. I'd go down to the building lobby (I lived in an apartment building then) to get the mail.

Toward the end of my second week at home, Karen told me it was time to go for a walk outside in the street. I was still using a walker, so it was pretty slow going. But just getting out into the real world again was a thrill in itself. And then there were the neighbors who had sympathetically observed my obviously painful efforts to get around in the weeks prior to surgery. Now they were all suitably impressed to see me on the move once again. And it sure massaged my ego to be told how brave I was.

That first day out I made it to the corner and back—maybe 100 yards total—but I could already see the new vistas that were opening up. My second time out, Karen showed me how to negotiate curbs:

Stepping off the curb, the walker goes first, then you step down with your operated leg and then your other leg. Up the curb, your walker goes first and then you step up with your good leg. Crutches work pretty much the same way except that going up a curb you don't put the crutches up first. It's all a matter of where the leverage is and keeping your balance.

My daily walk outside pretty quickly became one of the high points of my day. At first my wife would go with me, which was great just for the company; plus it gave me a chance to show off the progress I was making. But it was also reassuring in case I ran into difficulties, like the time I sat down on a bench that was too low and couldn't get up again.

One of the great things about walking is that it's a natural for short-term goals: the first time you go out in the street; the first time you go out in the street alone; the first time you walk up and down a curb by yourself; increasing your distance a block or two at a time. Each accomplishment merits a celebration, although you might want to save the Courvoisier for the red-letter days, like the first time I walked to our local coffee shop, about ten blocks away, had a cappuccino, and walked back all on my own! (I was using a cane by then.)

One way to motivate yourself to walk is by having a destination each time you go out. One day I'd walk to the park and watch the kids in the playground. Every bill I paid was another excuse to stroll down to the corner mailbox. Another day I'd walk to the library and browse through the new books or even the card catalog. Did we just run out of bananas? That was worth a trip to the local produce store.

Again, it's all a matter of attitude. I just love those people who refuse the role of invalid and create opportunities for their own therapy. Lady Andy from Los Angeles, for instance, writes:

Here's a tip for how to get some extra walking in. Go to the drugstore or market, and take a cart . . . you can use the cart like a walker, and go slowly up and down the aisles at your leisure. Mostly I just walk up and down, and don't buy anything. To rest, I stop at the prescription area where there are some chairs.

Doris Stokes of Fort Smith, Arkansas, walked most of the local mall while she was still using her walker. Two months after getting her new knee, she took a trip to Las Vegas and walked the strip. She also walked the length of both the Tulsa and Las Vegas airports. A few weeks later she went to Dallas for a Cowboys game and insisted on walking the mile from the parking lot to the stadium.

Swimming

Swimming is another great activity you can get back to—or start on—early. It isn't weight-bearing and it's very good cardiovascular exercise. But don't start until your doctor gives you the okay. He won't want you to start swimming until the staples have been removed and the wound is completely healed.

Of course, not everyone's a swimmer. But you really don't have to be. Just walking in the pool is good exercise because of the water resistance. And many pools and health clubs offer water aerobics classes, which are excellent. Just about any exercise in the water is good.

I learned how to swim as a kid, but for me swimming was more a fun way to cool off on a hot day than a sport I took seriously. When, as a result of my severe arthritis, I had to stop playing tennis and even walking was painful, swimming became my main physical activity. The first time I tried lap swimming, I barely managed two laps. After a month of swimming three times a week I was doing six to eight laps, and after two months I did a half mile (thirteen laps in my pool) every time.

In addition to swimming laps, I would get in a corner of the pool, hold on to the sides, and just kick up and down.

After a while I got fins, which, because they increased the resistance of the water while I was swimming, served as a knee-strengthening activity. But like many for whom swimming has not been a main sport of choice, I tended not to kick enough. So I hit on the idea of swimming every third lap on my back without using my arms, just kicking, as a way to concentrate on leg strengthening. The fins were great for this.

The biggest problem with swimming as an activity for joint-replacement patients is not the swimming itself but getting in and out of the pool. Your best bet, of course, is a pool with a set of graduated steps (many senior facilities have them). But I found after some cautious experimentation that I could ease myself into the water off the side of the pool and that I could pull myself up a ladder to get out.

Other Activities

An exercise bike is also very useful—especially on those days when you might not be able to go outdoors because of bad weather. In addition to being excellent exercise for the legs, pedaling a stationary bike is good for your general physical condition, especially the cardiovascular system. Most people requiring a joint replacement have been deconditioned for quite a while. In particular, the muscles around the joint have atrophied because they have not been used sufficiently.

But check with your physical therapist before you start. She will have some suggestions about when you're ready, how long to "ride" your bike, and especially the height of the seat. This last is important because the exercise bike can help in extending your knee flexion.

To help flexion you want to lower the seat to maximize

the stress on your knee. Then go back and forth on the pedals without making a complete rotation until you can comfortably go over the top. If you can do this with relative ease, lower the seat another notch until you can feel the pressure. If you can't make the rotation after several attempts, raise the seat a notch.

I started using my exercise bike this way about three weeks after my knee replacement. I'd usually do about five minutes with the seat at its low point and then raise it for easy cycling for another ten minutes. If you've had a hip replacement, don't lower the seat too much because you don't want your knee to go beyond a 90-degree angle with your torso.

Measuring Progress

How long will it take for me to get back to normal after my knee [or hip] replacement?" I always feel good when people ask me that question because it shows they have positive expectations about their surgery. Nevertheless, keep in mind there's no such thing as a one-size-fits-all answer. No two timetables are exactly the same. For one thing, what one person would find an acceptable level of "getting back to normal" might be totally unacceptable to another.

Your general physical condition is an important factor. If you're overweight, it will be more difficult to maintain an intense exercise level. Younger patients usually—but not always—recover sooner than older ones. But as I've said before and can't say often enough, the most important thing is your attitude.

When I asked Karen Sandy how a physical therapist measures a joint-replacement patient's progress, she replied:

We measure a person's progress in terms of function: how they're getting around, how they're doing their home activities of daily living, how they're managing the basics. I also measure their progress by how they're doing their exercises, how strong their leg seems to be getting.

Another way to measure progress is by measuring the patient's degree of flexion, range of motion, and degree of extension. I'll ask you to sit in a straight chair and, with your foot on the floor, bend your knee as far back as you can. This is a very objective way to let you know how you're doing. For instance, if you have 80 degrees of flexion, I'll tell you we're trying to get you to 90. A normal knee should be able to flex to around 130 degrees. The same with measuring your leg's extension. Full extension, when you can get your leg up absolutely straight, is measured as zero. Anything less than full extension is measured as a minus. These measurements are used to quantify progress as well as motivate someone to get further.

My progress was somewhat above average. When Karen first came to see me, my flexion measured 80 degrees and my extension minus 5. After three weeks of therapy, my flexion was at 100 degrees and my extension was minus 2.

Earlier we discussed the importance of short-term goals. But you also need what I call intermediate or turning-point goals such as switching from a walker (or crutches) to a cane.

Karen thinks that if you have a cemented joint you'll probably be able to go on to a cane—depending on how strong you are—within four to six weeks after surgery. But, she warns:

If you try to switch to a cane and you find you're limping or hopping, that means you can't weight-bear appropriately, so it's too soon. With an uncemented hip, it will usually be six weeks postop. That's when you'll have an X ray to assess the bone healing, and if it looks okay then the surgeon will usually say it's okay to try one crutch or a cane depending on how agile you are and how well you've progressed.

When you get to that point, your physical therapist will probably be ready to end your home visits. By then you'll be ready for the next stage: outpatient therapy.

CHAPTER 9

Tennis, Anyone?
Life After a Joint Replacement

What will my life be like after a joint replacement? Will I still have pain? What will I and won't I be able to do? How long will my prosthesis last? What if it has to be replaced?

If you're a prospective joint-replacement patient, these are undoubtedly among the main questions on your mind. The answers will not be the same for everyone. Even though knee and hip replacements have become almost routine, one key factor is still the skill and expertise of your surgeon. Other crucial factors in determining the level of success you'll achieve are your general health and the condition of your affected joint prior to surgery.

In addition, as I've said in the preceding chapter, the quality of your physical therapy and your commitment to it is critical to maximizing the extent of your recovery. Finally, as I've emphasized throughout these pages, your attitude—

especially the extent to which you take responsibility for your own rehabilitation—makes an enormous difference.

Although patients vary considerably in condition, general health, age, and attitude—and there *are* differences between surgeons and facilities—it is still possible to make a few generalizations that will apply to the vast majority of those getting new joints. To put it most succinctly, the quality of your life should be significantly better than it was prior to surgery, the pain should be substantially less, and you should be able to do a lot more than you would have been able to do without getting a replacement. This is the way it has worked out for most of us who have enjoyed the benefits of this young technology.

Once in a while, however, it doesn't work out that way. After her total knee replacement, writes Sally Pollock of Spanaway, Washington,

The pain kept increasing even with the 2400 mg of Motrin a day. I kept after my doctor, who put me in a weighted brace to force the leg to extend and bend more when I walked. He said I wasn't doing the exercises enough. It's a wonder he didn't break something when he pulled down with his weight to try to force my leg to straighten. Although the knee was twice the size of the other one, he told me not to worry, that it would eventually return to normal size.

After over eleven months of increasing agony, I convinced another doctor to listen to what I was saying. He finally opened my knee to see what was going on. It turns out the prosthesis was way too big, my shinbone was twisted 40 degrees, and my kneecap was positioned too low! Fortunately, my new doctor was able to replace the prosthesis with one that was the correct size so I can at least walk now, though with a slight limp.

Somewhere between four and six weeks after surgery, you will be at another critical turning point. Around that time, your surgeon will X-ray the area of your new joint to make sure everything is where it should be. By then you'll probably be able to drive yourself to your doctor's office. I did, and since it meant going from Oakland to San Francisco and back, it was my longest trip since leaving the hospital. Barring any unusual problems, you probably will not have to see your doctor again for at least another two months.

At this stage of your recovery, you should be able to get out of your house, shop for your basic needs, and get around in the street, probably using a cane. When you can do all that, the home visits of your physical therapist will come to an end. "Once you're able to get out of the house without too much pain or difficulty and you can manage it physically," says Karen Sandy, "I'm done."

But although your home therapist might be done, you're not. Of course, it would be wonderful if after six weeks, your remaining recovery could be accomplished without the grind of physical therapy. But this is when you'll need an extra shot of willpower. The temptation to ease up on your exercises and just let nature take its course will be strong. Big mistake! Although you've made good progress and you're starting to function on your own, you've still got a ways to go.

Remember that your body has gone through an extended trauma; not just the violence of invasive surgery but years in which your affected joint and the muscles and ligaments surrounding it were losing strength and deteriorating. You've put yourself through the duress of surgery in order to get your life back. You've already invested four to six weeks or so in physical therapy. So why sell yourself short now? That's the start of accommodating to a more circumscribed quality of life than is actually possible.

Donald Wray of Treasure Island, Florida, is a walking testament to the benefits of both joint replacements and an intensive program of postop therapy. Like me, Don is an avid tennis player—although I'm not in his class. (With his partner, he was ranked number one in Florida in doubles in the over-seventy division for four consecutive years.) But in 1996, approaching his seventy-fifth birthday, Don was forced to stop playing due to severe osteoarthritis.

Like me, Don was told that he would have to have both knees and one hip replaced. Wanting to get back to tennis as quickly as possible, he opted for a hip replacement in late October 1996 and bilateral knee replacements in early January 1997. All the operations were performed at Palms of Pasadena Hospital in St. Petersburg by Dr. Steven B. Warren. Don writes:

> Following hip surgery, I immediately started a five-day-a-week, two-hour-a-day physical therapy program at a nearby facility. I continued this until the day before I had my knees replaced. Following knee surgery I had physical therapy five days a week for five months and then tapered off to three days a week for a sixth month. I also did exercises at home.

A year later, Don was back with his old partner playing tournament tennis—now in the over-seventy-five class!

Outpatient Therapy

Almost everyone who has had a joint replacement will still need some kind of regular physical therapy after the home visits end. If you've had a knee replacement, you'll do best with the kind of supervised program you can get only at an outpatient facility. Hip-replacement patients also need continuing therapy, but they don't necessarily need the equipment you can only find at an outpatient facility.

Whether you've had a knee or a hip replaced, it's still a matter of attitude. There's not much point in going for outpatient therapy unless you make a serious commitment to a regular program plus a regimen of home exercises. The therapy you need for a hip replacement can, in most cases, be done at home. But without the regular supervision and monitoring of a therapist, you will have to be strongly motivated, so you might still consider outpatient therapy. Medicare covered my outpatient therapy for three months (three one-and-a-half-hour sessions a week). You'll have to check with your HMO.

In my case, I went for outpatient therapy after all three of my replacements—knees and hip—and I'm glad I did. Of course, my hip had been replaced so soon after my knees—five months between the second knee and the hip—that the therapy was probably as much for my knees as my hip. In fact, after the second knee replacement, I was forced to cut my outpatient therapy short because the pain from my hip was too acute to permit me to continue.

The big advantages of outpatient therapy—in addition to imposing regularity and consistency on your physical rehab—are the supervision and adjustment of your exercises and regular evaluations of your condition by the therapist. Plus an outpatient facility will have equipment you couldn't have at home.

Since your exercise regime will be individually tailored to your condition, there is no model program. What follows, therefore, is my own experience in outpatient therapy. But it will give you a general idea of what to expect.

.   .   .

Craig Norton has been a physical therapist for almost twenty-five years and directs the program for sports medicine rehabilitation at Cal-Sport, the Sports and Physical Therapy Center for Alta Bates Hospital in Oakland. That's where I went for my outpatient therapy, mostly because Karen Sandy had spoken so highly of Craig. I soon found out why.

By definition, therapists are hands-on people. But Craig is like a mother hen. He supervises a staff of about a dozen people who work with his patients, but he seems to be everywhere, seeing everything. He is also one of the shrewdest appraisers of his patients I've ever encountered—and, as you can imagine, I've seen more than my share of physical therapists.

Several years later, as I was working on this book, I went back to talk to Craig about his approach to physical therapy in general and sports medicine in particular. Here's some of what he said:

Basically, your physical therapist is a personal trainer with a medical background. He knows what you should do, what you can do, and what you should not do. Whether you've had a knee replacement, a shoulder replacement, a rotator cup repair, he has to know the protocols for each one. He needs to know your anatomy, your kinieseology, your pathology. But the therapist's job is really not hard. You don't have to be a rocket scientist. All he has to do is pull up those exercises he thinks will meet the patient's needs. The rest—and that's 90 percent of the program—really depends on the patient.

Above all, Craig is someone who loves sports and just about any form of physical exercise—and he manages to communicate this enthusiasm to his patients. As he puts it:

Whenever you exercise, you're working out at a level that's higher than your normal activities require. Any type of exercise is going to increase blood flow, it's going to increase bone density. It's just good for you. I just can't say that enough. That's the whole thing about exercise. Exercising is not just a physical thing. It's a philosophy. When you really exercise, it's body and mind and people don't understand that. People who never get into the mind part of exercising usually quit.

On my first visit, Craig gave me a thorough once-over, measuring my knee flexion and range of motion, testing my leg strength, and observing my gait and posture. "What I'll look for," says Craig, "is how you walk, how you look when you first walk into the facility. Then I look for swelling, range of motion, and pain. You can't get range of motion unless you get the swelling down. My objective is to build up your strength and give you a good gait, a good walking ability."

The results were everything I could ask for—and more. Four months after my hip replacement—the last of my three joint-replacement surgeries—when Craig first measured my range of motion, I had 102 degrees of flexion and minus 10 degrees of full extension on my left side. When I finished my final session almost three months later I had 110 degrees flexion and zero on the full extension. On the right side (where I had already made significant improvement because this was the side of my first knee replacement and because my hip replacement was on the left side), I started with zero on the extension and 122 degrees of flexion, and finished with zero and 127 degrees, respectively.

These may sound like small increments compared to the progress you'll probably make in the immediate postop period. (After getting home from the hospital I went from 80 to 100 degrees of flexion in about four weeks.) But those subsequent increments made an enormous difference in the level at which I was able function thereafter.

And it wasn't just the exercises. I valued Craig's personal attention, his constant monitoring, his encouragement, his enthusiasm, and his appropriate caution when I would get carried away by my usual eagerness to get on with my rehab.

Here's the way it worked:

Each session began with moist heat in the form of hot packs applied to the affected joints. (If you still have a lot of swelling you're more likely to get ice rather than heat.)

If you have a lot of pain, you might also be treated with what's called "interferential stim," in which low-level electrical impulses are sent into pads attached to the affected areas. The therapist will adjust these impulses to your tolerance level, giving you a buzz that you'll get to like after a while. (Craig says that some people even get addicted to it.)

I had the interferential stim after my knee replacements but didn't need it after my hip replacement.

The moist heat and the interferential stim are designed to make it easier for you to do the exercises by reducing pain and increasing mobility.

Exercises

Broadly speaking, your exercises are designed to do two things: increase your range of motion and strengthen your muscles. The two actually go hand in hand. As you get more range of motion you get better possibilities for gaining strength. Aside from the exercises using equipment, most were variations on those I had already been doing. But now they were done with weights or elastic bands (for resistance), the holds were longer, and there were more repetitions.

Thus, in Craig's version of the heel slide, I sat up on the massage table with my back against the wall and my legs straight out in front of me. An elastic band was placed under the sole of my foot and I would pull my leg gently upward, sliding my heel on the table, and then returning to the original position. I started off doing three sets of ten and gradually worked up to doing five sets of forty.

For the straight leg raise—an exercise for strengthening the thigh and hip muscles—I'd lie on my back, resting my upper body on my forearms, with my unoperated leg slightly bent. Then, keeping the knee locked, I'd lift the operated leg eight to ten inches off the table, hold that position for five seconds, and then lower the leg. I started out with three sets of ten, gradually increasing to five sets of twenty. After a week, ankle weights were added (first one pound and then two pounds).

Another good one is the wall slide. Standing flush against an unobstructed wall, I would slowly slide down six to eight

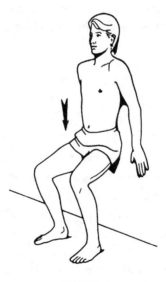

© VHI 1990

Wall Slide

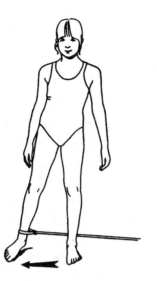

© VHI 1990

inches and then straighten up. I would do this thirty times, taking a few seconds' break after ten and then twenty.

Then there was a whole set of standing exercises using an elastic band and weights. The band would run around the leg of the massage table and then around my leg at the ankle. Craig used various colored bands, each color identifying a different level of resistance. First I would pull my leg away from the table and then bring it back. Then I would face away from the table and pull my leg forward. Then I would face the table and pull my leg back. And so on. By the time my outpatient therapy was finished, I was doing these in three sets of twenty-five each, for a total of seventy-five, with a five-pound weight.

Another excellent range-of-motion exercise uses a stationary bike. "One of the beauties of a stationary bike," says Dr. Susan Hochs, "is that there is no weight across the knee, unlike walking, jogging, etc. If the range of motion is good, biking is wonderful exercise during the rehabilitation period after a total knee replacement."

But don't just get on your bike and start pedaling. Your therapist should figure out the height of the seat, which usually will be lower than what it would be if you were riding outdoors, the idea being to increase the bend in your knee. In fact, the first few times I was on the bike, I couldn't even get a full rotation. Craig just told me to go as far as I could and then pedal back. The session when I could first turn the wheel over completely was one of those red-letter days for me.

One of the main features of an outpatient facility, of course, is the equipment. I got a big kick out of one called "the shuttle." It's a bit like a rowing machine except it's only for your legs. You lie down on a platform that is on a track, allowing the platform to move back and forth. Then, placing your feet against a vertical barrier, you push back and then return. The machine also has a resistance control so that as you progress, you'll be pushing harder. The fun part is that you're actually doing non-weight-bearing squats. This encourages your range of motion while improving the overall strength in your legs.

There were three other pieces of equipment at Cal-Sport that I used regularly. The orthotron is an apparatus you sit on with one or both feet in stirrups. Its purpose is to build your quadriceps and your hamstrings. You raise and lower your leg against pneumatic resistance at various rates of speed.

The eagle extension is somewhat similar. Sitting in a chair with a bar across your legs slightly above your ankles, you raise your legs, hold, and then lower them. As you get stronger, both the weight of the bar and the number of lifts are increased. You'll really feel this one.

On the eagle flex, you lie on your stomach with a weighted and padded bar across the back of your legs just above the Achilles tendon. This is also a lifting and lowering exercise. With this one you'll discover some muscles you didn't know you had.

There are dozens of variations on these exercises and others, and what your therapist programs for you might be different from what I did. At the end of your session you'll be cooled down with ice packs on your joints. If you have some swelling, you might be given treatment with high-galvanic stim—similar to interferential stim—which activates the large muscles around the joint. This in turn stimulates the veins to push the fluid back toward the heart (venous return).

Most of these programs are "progressive." That is, they are regularly increased, first by repetitions and then by resistance (weights or elastic bands). First the number of repetitions is increased. When the resistance is increased, the repetitions are dropped down and are then built back up again. According to Craig, this method will help keep you from pulling a muscle or a tendon.

To maximize the benefits of outpatient therapy, you should also be following a program of exercises at home. Remember, you're only going to outpatient therapy two or three times a week. You also must exercise on the days you don't go. Craig's advice was to do the same exercises—other than those that required the heavy equipment, of course—that I was doing at the facility. He gave me a set of elastic bands for that purpose, and I tried to do two half-hour sessions a day at home. If I did only one, I'd also do a half hour on the stationary bike my wife got me after my first arthroscopic surgery.

When your outpatient therapy has been completed, your next challenge is to incorporate a regular program of physical activity into your life. For people like myself who can't wait to resume their favorite sport, that's no problem.

But many people are not used to regular exercise. For whatever reason, they have never become attached to some sport or other physical activity they enjoy and to which they are committed. If you're one of those people, this is the time to change.

Sports: Do's and Don'ts

The easiest and most natural activity is walking. It's also one of the best things you can do—both for a replaced joint and for general health. In chapter 8 we discussed walking in terms of short-term rehabilitation goals. Now it's time to think about walking as a form of exercise over the long term.

Let's face it. Most people in our automobile-dependent society don't walk enough. We take the car for everything—even for trips to a store that's only a few blocks away. You can start by breaking the car habit. Even if you were to replace one automotive errand a day with a trip on foot you would have a good start on a regular exercise program.

Walking can be fun. It will help you to relate more directly to your neighborhood (and your neighbors), to your natural surroundings, and to new places you might visit. The important thing is to think about it as your sport, something that is both good for you and enjoyable. Plan on interesting places to go for walks. Most cities have pedestrian paths in parks, near lakes, or in nearby wooded areas. Your local parks department can probably send you a list of these. Walk around the local mall once a week.

Aim for a minimum of one mile a day. If you keep finding new and interesting places to walk, you'll do more.

Another good way to develop and maintain an exercise program is by joining a health club. Check out a few before signing up. There's a big range in rates, but some very good clubs are at the lower end of the scale. Many Y's have health facilities. Talk to your physical therapist about which exercises will be most beneficial and which to avoid.

Swimming is an excellent sport that will serve you well throughout your life. It is also a year-round sport if you have access to an indoor pool.

If you're not a swimmer, it's never too late to learn. Even if you don't swim, you can still exercise in the water. The good thing about water exercises is that they are non-weight-bearing, even though the water provides natural resistance that adds to the strengthening effects. Many facilities have senior swim hours, and if you can find one that also offers water exercise classes, you'll probably be allowed in no matter what your age. Many chapters of the Arthritis Foundation (check your local phone book) offer water-exercise classes especially designed for people with arthritis.

If you can swim—or if you are willing to learn—lap swimming is a terrific exercise with immense cardiovascular benefits—besides being tailor-made for those of us with joint replacements. My biggest problem with swimming is that I tend to find it boring, so for me it's more of a chore than the sports I usually associate with fun.

But my wife, who took up swimming only in her late fifties, derives great pleasure from it and has made it her main form of physical activity. She has become a regular lap swimmer, doing a minimum of a mile at least three times a week. She has what I can only describe as a kind of Zen attitude toward swimming; she uses it as a mind-cleansing process as well as physical therapy. Sometimes she concentrates on feeling her muscles working; other times on the rhythm of her strokes. Or else she makes it a time of reveries and mental pleasures, focusing on cloud formations (when she's doing a backstroke) or recalling the aroma of plants and trees.

Of course, some people are physically limited in what they can do. People with rheumatoid arthritis, for instance, often are not able to do things that most people—including those of us with osteoarthritis—take for granted. But they can still find a way to exercise regularly.

Forty-eight-year-old Robert Walters of Toronto, on a disability pension due to the ravages of rheumatoid arthritis, writes:

> With multiple prosthetics and rheumatoid arthritis I don't get the exercise a normal person gets from daily living. I have a set routine set up by a physiotherapist to maintain both my range of motion and my muscle tone. Also I attend "Arthritis classes" put on by my local Arthritis Society in heated therapy pools. Several times I have neglected doing these exercises for extended periods and have paid for it with loss of range or loose joints that are prone to injury.

Do not let the fact that you've had a knee or hip replacement discourage you from active sports. To the contrary, you now need regular, consistent physical activity more than ever—not just for your rehabilitation but for your general health, especially as you get older. The great advantage of finding a sport you enjoy is that you will be motivated to keep at it. I'm now playing tennis (doubles only) four times a week, and not only do I look forward to it, I plan the rest of my schedule around it.

Of course, not every sport is suitable for those who have had joint replacements. Football, for instance, is not a good idea. Neither is jogging. The following guide to post–joint-replacement sports activity is based on conversations with physical therapists, sports medicine doctors, orthopedic surgeons, and many patients. It's just a guide, but it might help you choose.

Avoid: racquetball, basketball, volleyball, soccer, tennis (singles)

Borderline: roller-skating, downhill skiing, tennis (doubles), mountain climbing

Use caution: outdoor bicycling, horseback riding, ice skating, hiking

Good to excellent: walking, swimming, golf, square dancing, bowling, cross-county skiing, ballroom dancing

My favorite physical activity—in case you haven't noticed by now—is tennis. Joint pain forced me to stop playing before my first knee replacement, and the desire to be able to play again was a big factor in my decision to go ahead with all three joint replacements.

You can see from the guide above that tennis is not among the highly recommended activities. Singles is in the "avoid" category because it inevitably involves a lot of running, and especially sudden twists and turns. As for doubles, I'd suggest you ask your doctor. That's what I did.

Dr. Wolf's response was: "I know that's one of your big-time goals. So I won't tell you not to do it. But you've got to be sensible about it." And that's what I try to do. I hardly ever play singles, and on the rare occasions when I do, I try to curb my competitive instincts. Mostly I play doubles. And I don't play every day; my limit is generally three or four times a week, and I usually avoid playing two days in a row. And I don't try to run down every single shot. (I couldn't even if I wanted to.)

Of course, I don't have the mobility I once did. But I'm able to cover more court than when I first started playing again. When I first got back on the courts, I could only return a ball that came within six feet. My playing partners were pretty nice about it, but I felt a lot like the kid who was always the last one picked when we were choosing up sides.

Now I'm a lot more mobile. I can even get to a lob hit over my partner's head about half the time, which I find pretty amazing—as do my opponents—and I'm no longer the last kid picked.

Daily Life

There is every reason to expect that you will be able to resume a normal daily life after your knee or hip replacement. How soon that will occur depends on many factors, however. People have different recovery times. Their general health conditions vary, as do their daily living circumstances.

Getting back to a normal daily routine at home will be a gradual process. The main thing is to get out of the invalid mode as quickly as possible. This will free you to try different things every day. Don't become frustrated with your limitations; learn to value the progress you're making. In time, you should be able to do nearly everything you used to do before your arthritis became symptomatic.

I felt comfortable with going out of the house by myself after about four weeks and with driving after about six weeks. Tennis took much longer. And some limitations will be permanent. (At age seventy-two, I wouldn't expect to be doing everything I did at thirty-two—or even at fifty-two—anyway.) I usually feel more comfortable if, in going up or down stairs, there's a banister I can use for support. And if the stairs are steep, I find a banister essential. But if the stairs are low and deep, I can manage them even if I'm carrying a tray or a laundry basket.

I avoid couches and soft chairs without arms. I can get up from them if I have to, but it's a chore. I need grab bars when bathing in a sit-down tub.

I still have a certain amount of stiffness in my knees, and I probably always will. But I have no problem walking. If I'm going to do some sustained walking, however, I take along a cane just in case.

How Soon Can I Return to Work?

I f you have a job, your main concern is probably being able to go back to work. Again, a lot depends on your particular circumstances, especially what kind of work you do and how you get to your job. Working at home sitting in front of a computer, I was back at my desk in about three weeks, but only for an hour at a time at first. If you travel to a job or if your work involves physical exertion, it will take longer. If you've had a hip replacement, you probably should allow a minimum of six weeks before going back to work.

Most people, irrespective of whether they've had a knee or a hip replaced, should be able to return to work somewhere between eight and twelve weeks after surgery.

Theater, Movies, Concerts, Museums

O ne of my biggest frustrations in the months leading up to my joint replacements was the fact that I had to severely curtail going to the theater and other cultural events. Long staircases or even short stairs without banisters, seats with cramped space for my legs, and the jostling I experienced in crowded aisles and lobbies made going out to such places not only uncomfortable but scary.

This is still a problem for me. I love live theater, and whenever I go to New York (usually twice a year to visit family) I make it a point to go to some shows. But I have learned the hard way that I have to be exacting in my choice of seats—especially in New York, where so many of the theaters were built with little attention to spacious seating.

Orchestra seats are the most expensive, but they're generally much better than mezzanine or balcony seats for those of us with joint replacements. Box seats with movable chairs are best, but they're also expensive and way on the side. For me—and this is true even today—an aisle seat that enables me to stretch out the stiffer of my legs is indispensable. (My wife and I are subscribers to two theater companies in the Bay Area, but a condition of our subscription was an aisle seat for me.)

If it's a show I absolutely must see, I take my chances on finding someone in a side aisle seat who would be willing to trade for my more centrally located spot. (Don't be bashful. People like to help.) On occasion I've gotten a friendly usher to let me sit on a chair off to the side or to take an empty seat in a box.

Movie houses—since most have been built more recently than theaters—are usually easier to manage. The aisles are wider, there tends to be more legroom, and only rarely do you have to deal with stairs. Even then I try to get an aisle seat, although I have rarely found a seat that wasn't manageable. Many movie houses these days also have special spaces for people in wheelchairs plus a seat alongside the space for a companion. If there's no one in one of those wheelchair spaces and the accompanying seat is not in use, however, you might be able to use the seat if you've got your handicap-parking permit (or some other document) showing that you've had a knee or hip replacement.

In both theaters and movie houses, balconies are treacherous. Most of them don't have handrails in the aisles, so walking down the stairs—especially if you're trying to do it when the houselights are off—is an adventure I could do without.

Although I do a fair amount of walking and play tennis, I have a hard time at museums. I'm all right for about half an hour, but after that my knees start imploring me to call it a day. But I'm not willing to give up museums. There are too many exciting shows and exhibits I want to see. Fortunately, more and more museums these days have wheelchairs for patrons who need them—and they're usually free or available for a very nominal charge. Not every museum has them, however, and if it's another one of those absolutely must-see exhibits (Picasso, Cézanne, the Impressionists) you might want to rent a wheelchair for the day. (Get a collapsible one, of course, so that you can put it in your car or in a cab.)

Travel

While you should be able to drive short distances without difficulty after four to six weeks, lengthier trips pose some problems. It will be many months before you'll feel comfortable either driving or just sitting in a car for eight hours—even if you're going to visit your grandchildren. That doesn't mean you shouldn't go. But it won't be a piece of cake.

I'd be cautious about taking a long trip for quite a while. If I did go, I wouldn't go alone. Instead, it would be with someone else who could do most of the driving. You'll find the trip much easier in the front passenger seat, where—with the seat pushed as far back as possible—you'll be able to stretch your legs to the maximum. No matter how it used to be, think of yourself as the relief driver who can take the wheel for short stretches of up to an hour. And it's a good idea—even when you're just a passenger—to take a ten-minute rest stop every hour in order to get out of the car and walk around a bit.

I'd avoid bus travel because the seats tend to be cramped and buses just aren't designed for getting up and walking around. Trains are much better since they have more legroom and it's much easier to get up and walk the aisles.

Of course, nothing beats planes for long-distance travel. This can be done, but it will take some planning. First, if you've got frequent-flyer miles that entitle you to upgrades to first class or connoisseur class, this is the time to use them. You'll still want to get up and walk around often, but if, like most of us, you're used to flying coach, the wide seats and spacious legroom will be bliss.

If you must fly coach, ask for one of those seats with extra space in front. These are often at emergency exits, and the airline might be reluctant to have you sit there, but if you have a traveling companion who can sit next to the exit door while you occupy the aisle seat, the airline might go for it. Otherwise, get an aisle seat, which will give you the maximum stretching room. Make sure it's on the side that will enable you to stretch your operated leg out into the aisle.

Finally, wherever you go, make sure you have some kind of ID documenting that you have a joint replacement. Your surgeon should be able to supply you with one. After my first knee replacement, Dr. Wolf gave me a letter on his stationery certifying that I had a replacement knee. After my hip replacement, he gave me a plastic card, issued by the manufacturer of my implant and certified by him as my surgeon, that says: "The owner of this card has a total joint replacement and has in place a permanent metal implant. This implant may activate a metal detection device."

Actually much to my disappointment, my new joints only triggered an airline metal detector once—although my keys and loose change have done so many times. But my card has helped me out in dozens of other situations. On a trip to Italy in the spring of 1997, for instance, it got me to the head of the line going into the Vatican Museum (usually a three-hour wait). So, as the ad says, "Don't leave home without it!"

What About Sex?

If you were sexually active before your joint replacements, you should definitely be able to resume a sex life afterward. "In fact," notes the *Total Hip Replacement Guide* of the Hospital for Special Surgery, "patients who, in the past, have had impaired sexual function caused by preoperative hip pain and stiffness usually find that, after surgery, their hips are pain-free and have better motion."

The real question is not whether but how—and when. As to how, especially in the first couple of months, it's pretty much the way porcupines make love: carefully! Hip-replacement patients should be particularly careful in light of the general restrictions they have to observe for the first six weeks. Both the Hospital for Special Surgery and the orthopedics department at the University of Iowa Hospitals advise hip-replacement patients to avoid sexual intercourse for four to six weeks. The rest really depends on what you and your partner can handle and what positions you feel most comfortable with. But this is no time for coyness. Talk over the details with your partner. Perhaps the following illustrations from the guidebook for hip-replacement patients offered by the Hospital for Special Surgery will make it easier to discuss.

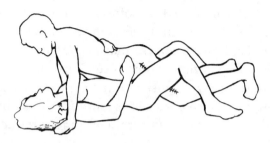

Patient on the top: partner on the bottom (and vice versa)

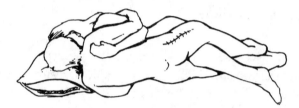

Patient lying on side with operated leg on top

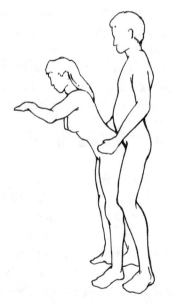

Standing position for both patient and partner

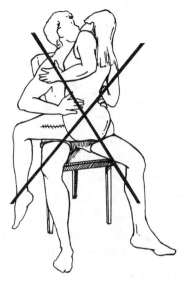

Too much hip abduction, flexion,
and rotation

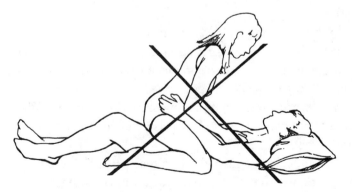

Too much hip flexion

One Good Joint Deserves Another

Once you've had a knee or a hip replaced, the odds increase that sooner or later your other knee or hip will also have to be replaced. After I was diagnosed with osteoarthritis and had X rays taken of all my key joints, I was told that I had "a lot of arthritis in my body" and that it was especially severe in both my knees and my hips. At the time, only my right knee was symptomatic. But once one of those joints gets really bad it seems to throw your other weight-bearing joints out of kilter. For instance, there have been studies showing that people with osteoarthritis of the knee compensate at the expense of the hip while getting out of a chair.

The other joints are also given extra duty during the immediate recovery period after replacement of the joint that's in the worst condition.

Both my left knee and my left hip became very painful about four months after my right knee was replaced, and it was a bit of a toss-up as to which would have to be replaced first. Dr. Wolf finally decided that the knee was giving me more problems than the hip, but five months after my left knee was replaced I was back on the operating table again for my left hip.

On the other hand, Dr. Wolf was pretty sure I'd need to have my other hip replaced fairly soon. But as I write this, it's four years since I had my left hip replaced and my right hip seems to be holding up well. I do get some low-level pain there once in a while, especially after playing tennis or extended walking, and it won't come as a total surprise if I need to have that one done sometime, too.

Roberta Suarez, a retired schoolteacher from Staten Island, New York, who has both osteoarthritis and rheumatoid arthritis, faced a similar situation. Both her knees and one hip were symptomatic. In her case, the hip was replaced first, the surgery performed by Dr. Thomas Sculco at the Hospital for Special Surgery in New York City on January 15, 1997. Despite the other problems, her recovery went very well, so much so that by the time she was discharged from the hospital, she writes: "I was able to walk with a cane and up the steps when I got home." And, she adds, "I was never in any pain, just a little stiff until the new joint worked itself in."

Six months later, Roberta's left knee was replaced by the same surgeon at the same hospital. Although a double knee replacement was considered, Dr. Sculco decided against it because the right knee was not as bad as the left. Again, her recovery was excellent. After a week in the hospital and another week in a rehab unit, Roberta was able to go from a walker to a cane to walking without any aid at all. And, as of this writing, replacement of her other knee has been put off indefinitely.

This doesn't mean that you're inevitably slated for a series of joint replacements. I know many people who have had just one joint replaced. I know quite a few others who have had both knees or both hips replaced—and that's all. The number with three joint replacements is significantly less, and even fewer have gone bionic in all four.

All of which is to say that it's best to be prepared. I don't use a cane or a walker anymore, but I've still got both—as well as my raised toilet seat and the various gadgets I used in the early stages of recovery. I hope I never need them again, but they're stored away where I can get to them easily just in case. It's also important to be prepared psychologically. I hope you won't need more joint replacements. But if you do you will have the advantage of knowing what to expect and that the pain and frustration you're suffering will come to an end.

How Long Will a Joint Replacement Last?

One of the main considerations that come up in every discussion of joint replacements is how long they will last. When I was told, at the age of sixty-seven, that I was "too young" for a total knee replacement, it was because of concern that I was likely to outlive my new joint. I would therefore require a second replacement which would be a much more complex operation with a lower success rate.

No one knows for sure how long a prosthesis will last. Most doctors will tell you that the life expectancy of a new knee or a new hip is ten to fifteen years. But that ballpark figure was arrived at some time ago, before extensive experience with the newer prostheses had been accumulated.

Since modern joint-replacement surgery is still very young, however, there haven't been that many statistical studies on prosthetic life expectancy. A recent study of hip replacements by Dr. John J. Callaghan, head of orthopedics at the University of Iowa Hospitals and Clinics and one of the top orthopedic surgeons in the country, suggests that the prevalent estimate needs significant upward revision:

Total hip arthroplasty has been performed for approximately 25 years in the U.S. with over 100,000 procedures performed annually. Pain relief is excellent, with over 95% of patients obtaining 90–95% relief of the pain caused by hip arthritis, and is maintained over 20 years in the majority of patients. In addition, high functional level is maintained. Fifty percent of patients I study performed at least light labor at 20 years follow-up, including maintaining a home, performing house cleaning, and mowing the lawn. . . . *Eighty-five percent of patients alive at a*

minimum of 20 years of follow-up still retained their orig-
inal hip replacement (emphasis added). (*Journal of the*
American Medical Association, August 1996)

The current techniques and prostheses used in knee
replacements are so new that statistics on them are not yet
available. But orthopedic surgeon Dr. Paul Lotke, at the Hospital of the University of Pennsylvania in Philadelphia, says:
"A good total knee replacement will never feel as normal as a
good total hip replacement, but it will last longer. In fact, 97
percent of knees implanted will still be kicking, so to speak,
ten years after surgery, and 92 percent twenty years after
surgery." (*Modern Maturity*, September–October 1997)

A long-term study of more than 100 total-knee-replace-
ment patients under the age of fifty-five by a group of doctors
at the Insall–Scott-Kelly Institute for Orthopaedics and
Sports Medicine at the Beth Israel North Medical Center in
New York City—believed to be the largest such study ever
made—concluded: "With failure defined as revision of either
the femoral or the tibial component, the overall rate of survival [of the prosthesis] was 94 percent at eighteen years."
The doctors deliberately focused on younger patients
because of the widespread concern that such patients might
have to undergo numerous revisions in the course of a lifetime. ("Total Knee Replacement in Young, Active Patients:
Long-Term Follow-up and Functional Outcome"; *Journal of
Bone and Joint Surgery*, April 1997)

The chief cause of failure in a joint replacement is loosening of the prosthesis. The main reason for this is that the
bones that make up a normal joint are living organisms and
the prosthesis is not. Consequently, your body cannot regenerate the components of a prosthesis as, over time, it starts to
loosen and break down. Or, as Dr. Wolf puts it:

There are two cells in bone. There are cells that destroy bone and cells that produce bone. So what you have is a constant process of renovation. Bone being destroyed and right behind it, bone being rebuilt. Just going through daily life, your body is under such stresses and strains that you need to constantly rebuild it. Therefore, a total joint can't ever replace the normal joint. Because there are no maintenance engineers there rebuilding it as it breaks down.

Revisions

When a joint replacement breaks down, it is possible, in most cases, to put in a new one. But these "revisions"—as orthopedic surgeons call them—tend to be more difficult and somewhat less successful than first-time replacements.

Revision is a different, more complicated operation. First the surgeon has to take out the cement (if it was previously used), which is quite difficult. Then the old prosthesis has to be removed and the joint reconstructed again. This time the surgeon will need additional hardware and new stabilizing structures. New bone grafts might be needed, and the prosthesis might not be the same. Consequently, the operation takes much longer. I have heard of cases where a patient getting a revision was on the operating table for as long as eight hours. "Any time you do a second operation," says Dr. Wolf, "the difficulties increase, the complications increase, recovery becomes more difficult, and the results are not as good." This is the main reason surgeons urge people to put off a total joint replacement as long as possible.

Not all revisions are total, however. Donald Walden, a

retired electrician, had a total knee replacement in May 1995 at the Kaiser Hospital in Sacramento. Two years later he had a fall injuring the same knee. X rays showed that the prosthesis had loosened where it was cemented into the lower leg bone. In October 1997 he went back to Kaiser, where the original surgeon, Dr. Plemmons, did the revision. It turned out that only the lower portion of the prosthesis had to be replaced. Still, the operation took five hours.

Three weeks later, Don wrote to tell me he was finding "the recovery faster and a lot less painful than it was the first go-round. I can walk upstairs without a cane, almost without a limp. I carry a cane but don't use it much."

Not everyone can have a revision. It all depends on the available bone. People with osteoporosis, for instance, often have so little bone left that a revision operation becomes impossible. (Sometimes they are unable to have even the first replacement.)

On the other hand, younger patients and people with good bone structure might be able to have several revisions to the same joint. There's no reason to be reckless after a joint replacement, but I've heard of people who wore out three and four knee replacements by dancing and younger patients with as many as four revisions on the same hip.

. . .

The science—or "art," as Dr. Wolf prefers to call it—of joint replacement is still very new. Almost every year brings improvements in surgical technique, prosthesis design, materials, and the rehabilitation processes. As a result of these innovations and the accumulated experience of several million knee and hip replacements, the success rate has been climbing, prostheses are lasting longer, and recoveries are becoming more complete.

Another exciting development is that knees and hips—although they are the most widely done—are not the only joints being replaced. More and more shoulders are being replaced, and attempts are now being made to develop effective ankle, elbow, wrist, and finger joint replacements.

But beyond the statistics, the surgery, the doctors, and the therapy are the patients—the real point of all medicine.

For me, not a day goes by that I don't thank my lucky stars that I can walk out my front door, pick up my morning paper, play with my grandchildren, go out to dinner or to the movies without having to think twice about it, play tennis, and look forward to years of the same—all because dedicated doctors, physical therapists, and other professionals were determined to make it possible for people like me to have normal, productive, pain-free lives again.

What's truly amazing—and inspiring—however, is that there are hundreds of thousands of people (maybe millions by now) just like me, who probably start off every day saying much the same thing.